GW01377186

THE SOUS VIDE FORMULA BOOK

A Collection of the Best 2021's Sous Vide Recipes for Taking the First Step in a New Way of Experience Food

Sous Vide Secrets

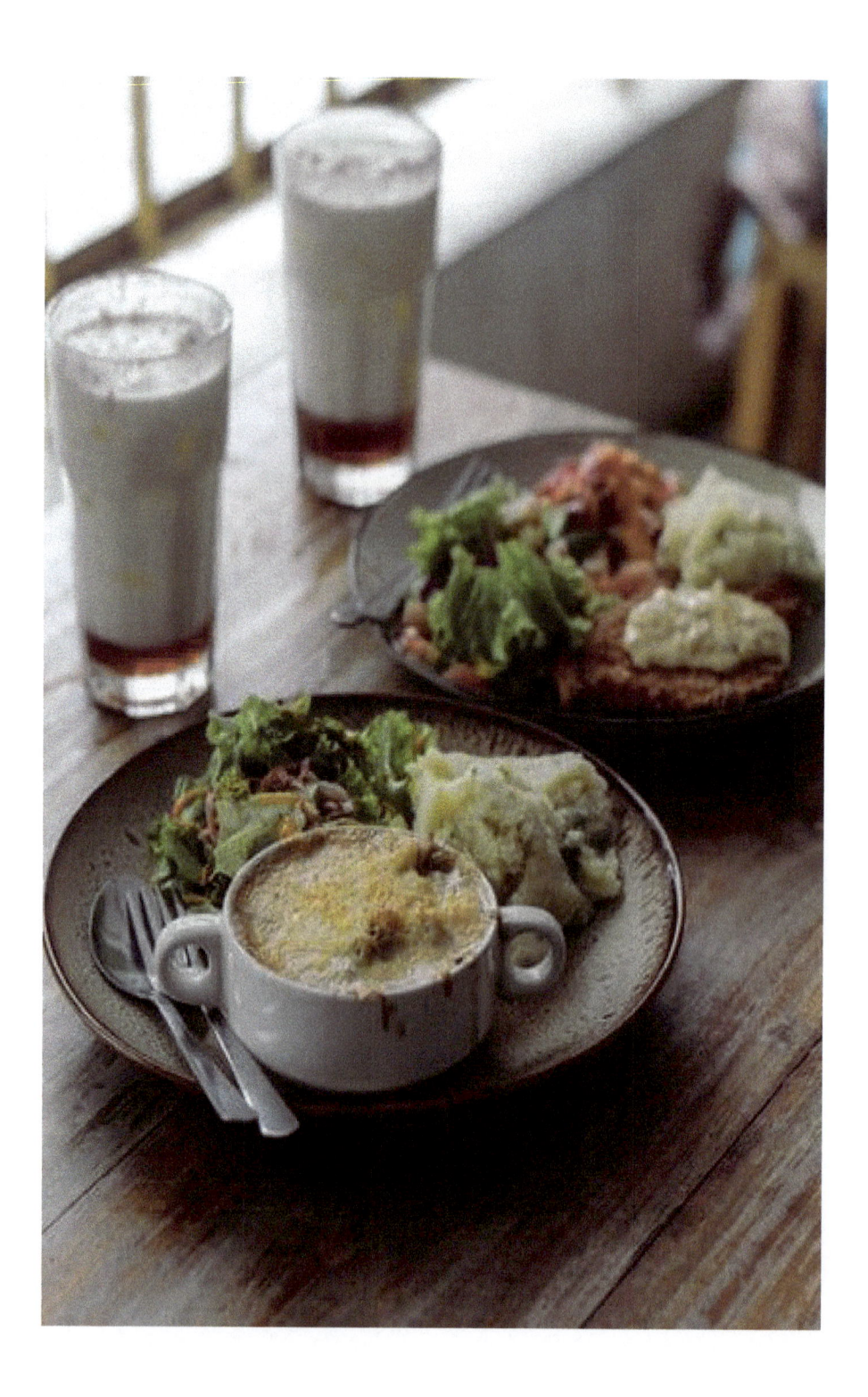

© Copyright 2021 by Sous Vide Secrets - All rights reserved.

The following Book is reproduced below to provide information that is as accurate and reliable as possible. Regardless, purchasing this Book can be seen as consent to the fact that both the publisher and the author of this book are in no way experts on the topics discussed within and that any recommendations or suggestions that are made herein are for entertainment purposes only. Professionals should be consulted as needed before undertaking any of the actions endorsed herein.

This declaration is deemed fair and valid by both the American Bar Association and the Committee of Publishers Association and is legally binding throughout the United States.

Furthermore, the transmission, duplication, or reproduction of any of the following work including specific information will be considered an illegal act irrespective of if it is done electronically or in print. This extends to creating a secondary or tertiary copy of the work or a recorded copy and is only allowed with the express written consent from the Publisher. All additional rights reserved.

The information in the following pages is broadly considered a truthful and accurate account of facts and as such, any inattention, use, or misuse of the information in question by the reader will render any resulting actions solely under their purview. There are no scenarios in which the publisher or the original author of this work can be in any fashion deemed liable for any hardship or damages that may befall them after undertaking the information described herein.

Additionally, the information in the following pages is intended only for informational purposes and should thus be thought of as universal. As befitting its nature, it is presented without assurance regarding its prolonged validity or interim quality. Trademarks that are mentioned are done without written consent and can in no way be considered an endorsement from the trademark holder.

Table of Contents

INTRODUCTION 1

BREAKFAST 20

    Seeds Porridge 22

    Chicken and Eggs 23

    Chia Eggs and Lime 25

    Broccoli Eggs 26

    Ginger Tomatoes Eggs 27

    Bok Choy and Veggies Bowls 30

    Bok Choy and Eggs 32

    Greens and Eggs 33

    Eggs and Asparagus 34

COCKTAILS AND INFUSIONS 35

    Lavender Syrup 36

    Thyme Liqueur 38

    Vodka Lemon Meyer 39

Rosemary & Lemon Vodka 41

Bloody Mary Vodka 42

Coffee Liquor 44

Honey Ginger Shrub 46

Cherry Bourbon 48

Bacon Vodka 49

LUNCH 50

Peppers and Green Beans 52

Savory Oatmeal with Mushrooms 53

Spicy Kidney Beans 55

Delicious Lentil Curry 58

Fried Tofu in Peanut Sauce 60

Grand Marnier 62

Red Wine Plum Shrub 64

Lamb Shoulder 65

SNACKS 66

Bacon Brussels sprouts 68

Okra with Chili Yogurt 69

Sous Vide Ratatouille 71

Potato Salad 74

Rosemary Fava Beans 76

Thyme Lard Broad Beans 79

Tomato Confit 80

Pears in Pomegranate Juice 82

DINNER 84

Crab Zucchini Roulade with Mousse 85

Herbed Prawns 88

Elk Steak 90

Lamb Steaks 93

Lamb Sweetbreads 95

Venison Steaks 97

Osso Buco 101

Rabbit Loin 104

DESSERT 106

Vanilla Apricot Crumble 108

Savory Banana & Nuts Cups 109

Orange Cheesy Mousse 111

Coconut Blackberry Tart 114

Lemon & Berry Mousse 116

Creamy Blueberry Mousse 118

Fruity Chocolate Flan 120

Maple Lemon Brioche Pudding 123

INTRODUCTION

We all enjoy quality food. Foodies often travel many miles to explore and get a taste of fantastic cuisine from all around the world.

For most of us, though, it is not possible to sample such delicacies, perhaps due to lack of time, money, or experience to prepare the meals ourselves.

In the past, the only option would be to save money and take a vacation to a place with gourmet food.

But things have changed, thanks to the fact that sous vide circulators are now available at an affordable price.

While there are some pretty fantastic new cooking appliances such as the air fryer, Instant Pot, crock pot, etc., sous vide circulators are in a league of their own.

The best part of sous vide, you ask?

Regardless of the level of your experience, you will be able to prepare a perfect meal every single time!

This may seem hard to believe at first, but it's true.

Before exploring the more than 500 fabulous recipes in this book, I would ask you to walk through this in-depth introductory chapter that will introduce you to the basics of Sous Vide cooking and help you master the art.

This book is targeted toward amateurs and new chefs alike, so everything is broken down into easy to understand sections.

History of Sous Vide Cooking

Generally speaking, the process of vacuum sealing food to extend shelf life has been around for a long time. However, it didn't gain recognition as a cooking method before the 1940s. Even after that, it took a lot of experimentation before people started to place vacuum-sealed food in a pot full of boiling water to cook it!

As a cooking method, the origin of the sous vide technique, therefore, finds its roots in the mid-1970s, when Chef Georges Praulus tried to develop a cooking technology that would minimize costly shrinkage and help create an optimal cooking environment for cooking foie gras.

The technique of sous vide cooking was not confined to him. Soon after Praulus introduced the technique to the world, Chef Bruno Goussault took up the method and refined it further, which allowed him to use sous vide to craft meals for the first-class travelers of Air France.

Seeing the hidden potential behind the technique, Bruno worked relentlessly to bring the method to the mainstream market.

However, despite reaching mass popularity, it was still too costly for ordinary people to afford, and it took two more years of evolution before it completely broke through to become one of the best cooking techniques ever developed.

Contrary to popular belief, thanks to a large number of affordable sous vide circulators available in the market, anyone can pick up the device and start experimenting with sous vide cooking!

The Science behind Sous Vide Cooking

Despite having become very popular, the sous vide cooking technique still creates confusion among beginners.

Let me help you clarify the concept a bit.

Let's start with the fundamental element first:

What exactly does "sous vide" mean?

The term "sous vide" is French for "under vacuum."

The name itself is inspired by the process that is used in sous vide cooking.

Perhaps one of the major differences between sous vide and other traditional cooking methods is that in sous vide, you will put all of your ingredients to either a Ziplock bag or in a Mason jar and seal them up in such a way that a vacuum is created inside.

This sealed vessel is then submerged under water that is heated to a certain temperature with utmost precision using the sous vide circulator, which allows for perfect cooking every single time.

The whole process greatly simplifies cooking—even for amateurs—and allows anyone to create masterpieces in no time.

Advantages of Sous Vide

While the above-mentioned advantages focus on the general aspects of sous vide, the following will provide you an elaborate outline of the health benefits of sous vide.

- While cooking with sous vide devices, you won't need to add any kind of additional fats needed in other methods. This immediately eliminates the need for using harmful oils that increase the cholesterol levels of the food, making sous vide meals much healthier.
- Exposing ingredients to heat, oxygen, and water causes them to lose a lot of vital nutrients, leading to over-carbonization of meats and vitamin/antioxidant loss in vegetables. The vacuum sealing technique that is implemented while cooking with sous vide prevents this from happening, as the food is not exposed to any water or oxygen. As a result, the nutritional contents are preserved to near-perfect levels.
- Sous vide cooked meals are easier to digest, as it helps to break down the collagen proteins into gelatin, which is easier for our body to digest and absorb.

- Undercooking is very harmful, as it not only leads to unpleasant tasting food but also leaves in bacteria and viruses. The vacuum seal of sous vide prevents this from happening, and the oxygen that is required for the pathogens to live is sucked out. The precise cooking technique ensures that you are getting perfectly cooked meals every single time.

Essential Kitchen Equipment

As mentioned before, there is a very common misconception among people who think that sous vide cooking requires a lot of expensive equipment and appliances.

While it is true that expensive equipment is available that would allow you to create even more "premium" meals, it is still possible to achieve the same level of satisfaction without emptying your bank account.

Thanks to technological advancements, sous vide circulators have become very cheap and affordable (you can get some good ones for as low as 60$!), which makes it easier to try sous vide cooking.

Aside from the circulator itself, you need a few other pieces of equipment, which are easily available for low prices in the supermarket or can even be found at your home!

I will be talking about all of them in a bit, but, before that, let me talk a bit about the sous vide circulator itself.

The Sous Vide Immersion Circulator

Sous vide circulators are the heart of sous vide cooking.

The main purpose of these devices is to simply heat up your water bath to a very specific temperature with utmost precision and maintain that specified temperature throughout the cooking process.

The circulator also circulates the water to ensure that the heat is distributed evenly.

If you are buying a sous vide circulator for the first time, though, the following are the best ones available right now.

- **Anova Precision Cooker with Wifi:** The Anova Wifi circulator is the top dog in the sous vide business, and it took the world by storm when it launched. Aside from the obvious cooking functionality, other additional features like Bluetooth or WiFi connectivity that allows for wireless controlling makes this the complete package, perfect for beginners!

    At the time of writing, the lowest market price was $109.

- **ChefSteps Joule:** While Anova is considered the leading device, the ChefSteps Joule is the pioneer when it comes to the "smart kitchen" scene. Back when this device was introduced, aficionados instantly fell in love with the device, thanks to its compact size and robust array of features.

At the time of writing, the lowest market price was $199.

- **Gourmia Sous Vide Pod:** The Gourmia is the one to go for if you are on a tight budget. This Sous Vide circulator has all of the basic functionalities that you would expect without sacrificing aesthetics.

At the time of writing, the lowest market price was $59.

Aside from the circulator itself, the following are some other essential items.

- A reasonably large container

You are going to need a good quality container to prepare your water bath in order to submerge your vacuum-sealed container and cook the contents. Therefore, it is wise to go for a good quality 8-12-quart stockpot. However, if that is not possible, then you should go for a 12-quart square, polycarbonate food storage container, just to be safe. Either way, make sure to purchase a container that has the capacity to hold water heated to 203 degrees Fahrenheit.

- Resealable bags and jars

Once you are set with the container, the next items you are going to need are the resealable bags and sealing jars.

When considering the bags, you should go for heavy-duty, resealable bags that are capable of sustaining a temperature of up to 195 degrees Fahrenheit. If possible, get bags that are marked "freezer safe" and come with a double seal.

For the jars, simply go for Mason jars or canning jars that come with a tight lid.

You might notice that throughout the book we used the "immersion" method for sealing zipper bags and "finger tight" techniques for tightening cans; both of the techniques are explained below.

- Cast Iron Pan

Some recipes will ask you to sear your meal after sous vide cooking is done, so keeping a cast iron pan nearby is a good decision.

Alternatively, you may also achieve a brown texture using a blowtorch.

Basics of Sous Vide

While some recipes will call for deviations in the process, the following are the basic steps that you are to follow while cooking using your sous vide device.

Prepare: Once you have decided which container to use, simply attach the immersion circulator to the container and fill it up with water. Make sure to keep the height of the water just one inch above the minimum water mark of the circulator that you are using.

Dutch ovens, plastic storage containers, stockpot, and large saucepans are good options for sous vide cooking.

Choose temperature: Set the temperature of your circulator as asked by your recipe.

Pre-heat water bath: Turn the device on and allow the water bath to reach the desired temperature. It should take about 20-30 minutes, depending on your device.

Season and seal the meal: Season your food as instructed by the recipe and vacuum seal it in either zipper bag or canning jars.

Submerge underwater: Once the desired water level has been reached, and you have sealed your bags, submerge the food underwater and cover the container with a plastic wrap.

Wait until cooked: Wait until cooking is complete.

Add some finishing touches: Take your bag out and follow the remaining instructions for some finishing touches!

Getting to Know the Sealing Techniques

While you can most definitely use expensive devices to seal your zipper bags automatically, you may simply use the method described below to vacuum seal bags easily.

Water Immersion Method: This method is also sometimes known as the Archimedes principle method. The steps are as follows:

- Put the ingredients in your bag.
- Gently start to submerge the bag under water, making sure to keep the upper part (the enclosure) above water.
- As you keep on submerging the bag underwater, the pressure from the water will slowly push out all the air that may be present in the bag.
- Submerge it just up to the zipper and quickly close it, making sure that no water has entered the bag.
- That's it! Simple as that.

As for canning jars, the finger tight technique is what you need to know.

Finger Tight: The finger tight technique is used for tightening jars.

For this technique, all you have to do is tighten the lid of your jar gently and stop just at the moment you start to feel the slightest amount of resistance.

This is to ensure that the air is able to escape from the inside once you submerge the jar.

General Tips

- If you are planning on saving some time while prepping the foods, then you may purchase meats that are already sliced and cut in the shape that you prefer. Some stores even offer foods that are prepackaged in sous vide sealed plastic bags. Such meats are already prepared and can be put under a water bath without any further preparation.
- If you have a vacuum sealer, simply put the meat in a bowl with a brine solution and place it in the vacuum chamber. Turn the device on, and the vacuum sealer will pull all the air out of the meat, which will allow the marinade to instantly bond with the meat and fill in the gaps.
- Putting garlic in sous vide meals can often bring out a bitter flavor; to avoid this, try to look for a spice known as asafoetida. This particular spice comes from the same family as garlic and onions but does not infuse your meal with the bitter garlic taste.
- Sometimes, once you have sealed your meals either using the immersion method or a vacuum sealer, the edges might end up flat, which might distort the shape of some food. This can be tackled easily

by adding a flavorless oil, such as vegetable oil, to the bag before sealing it.

- Sous vide circulators might take a bit of time to heat up your water bath; to speed up the process, add already-heated water to your sous vide container, such as from a kettle or boiled on the stove, and place the sous vide circulator in afterward. This will allow the water to reach your specified temperature quickly.
- If you cook a lot of vegetables, there remains a possibility of developing brown edges from acid development. A good way to tackle this is to sprinkle a bit of baking soda on before sealing them.
- If the recipe requires you to sear your food, you will be asked to use an extremely hot pan. To ensure that you're able to handle this safely, keep tongs close to your cooking station.
- Once you are done with sous vide cooking, make sure to fully dry your meat before searing, grilling, or torching it.

Sous Vide Food Safety Tips

Like all other cooking methods, sous vide cooking will also require you to handle and serve food in a safe manner to make sure that everything is perfect.

1. With any food, it is essential to cook the food long enough to ensure that foodborne pathogens are eliminated. Make sure to prepare the meals according to the specified temperature and for the specified period. However, if you are trying something new, then try to find your ingredient in the chart below and cook accordingly.
2. The safest way is to seal the food and put it directly in pre-heated water. However, when you seal the food in plastic, you should consider the temperature at which they are sealed and for how long you are going to store them. Sealing food creates an oxygen-free environment that allows anaerobic bacteria to grow. You may easily avoid this by making sure that meat and poultry are below 40 degrees Fahrenheit while you are sealing them, and seafood are frozen.
3. Cross-contamination of food is one of the major ways through which foodborne illness are spread; people often tend to handle uncooked meat, fish, or poultry in unsanitary conditions that lead to

contamination. The way to avoid this is to have a completely sanitized cooking station and make sure that the surface and cooking utensils are properly washed with hot water or a chlorine solution.

BREAKFAST

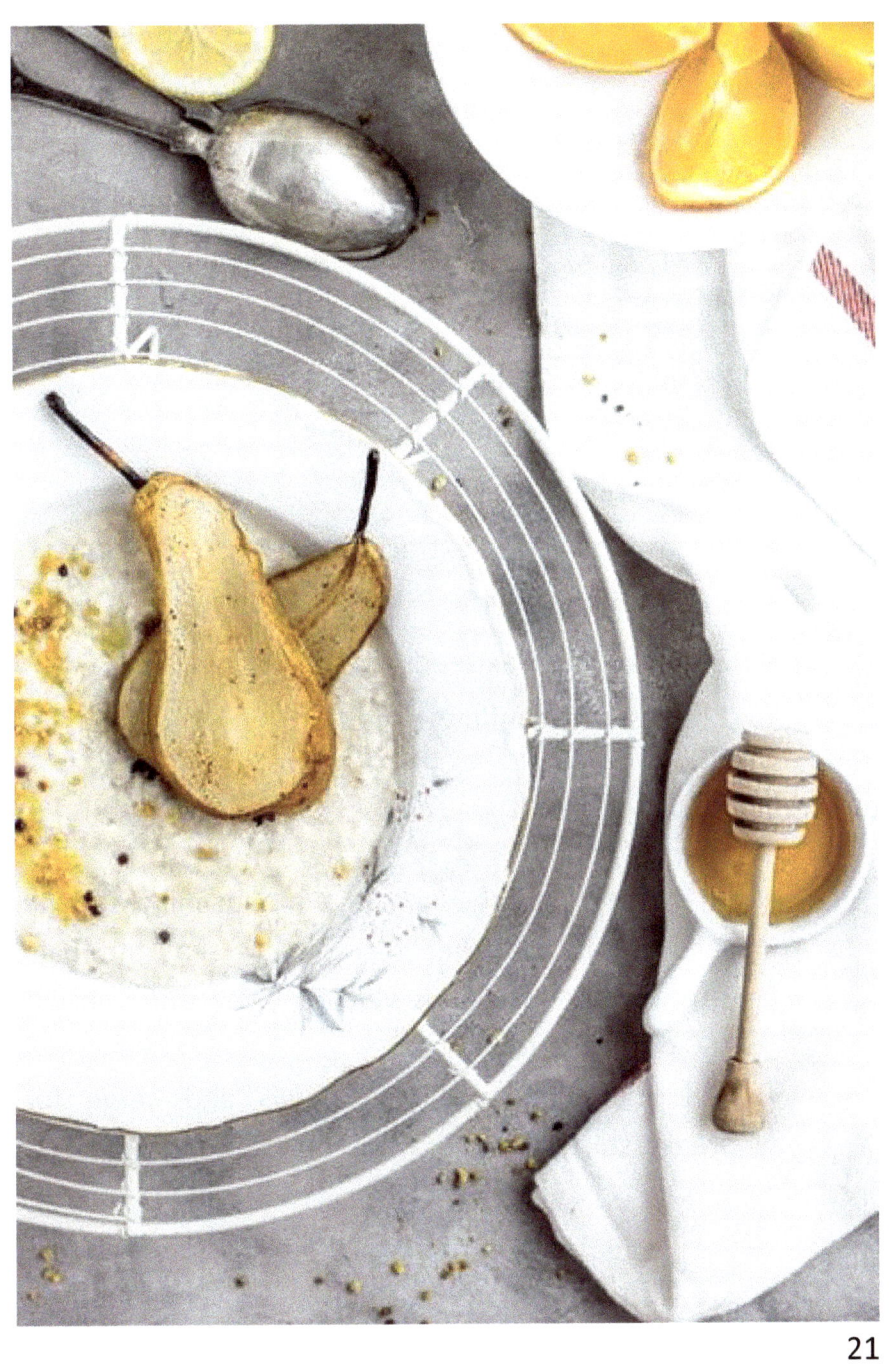

Seeds Porridge

2 Servings

Preparation time: 1 hour 3 minutes

Ingredients:

- ½ cup heavy cream
- ½ teaspoon cinnamon powder
- 1 tablespoon sugar
- ¾ teaspoon vanilla extract
- 1 cup almond milk
- 2 tablespoons flax seeds
- 1 tablespoon sunflower seeds

Directions:

- In a sous vide bag, mix the almond milk with the seeds and the other ingredients, seal the bag, introduce in your sous vide machine and cook at 180 degrees F for 1 hour
- Divide the porridge into bowls and serve for breakfast.

Chicken and Eggs

2 Servings

Preparation time: 40 minutes

Ingredients:

- 4 eggs, whisked
- 1 avocado, peeled, pitted and cubed
- Salt and black pepper to the taste
- 1 cup rotisserie chicken, cooked and shredded
- ½ cup black olives, pitted and halved
- 1 tomato, chopped

Directions:

- In a sous vide bag, combine the meat with the eggs and the other ingredients, toss, seal the bag, introduce in your sous vide machine and cook at 170 degrees F for 30 minutes.
- Divide between plates and serve.

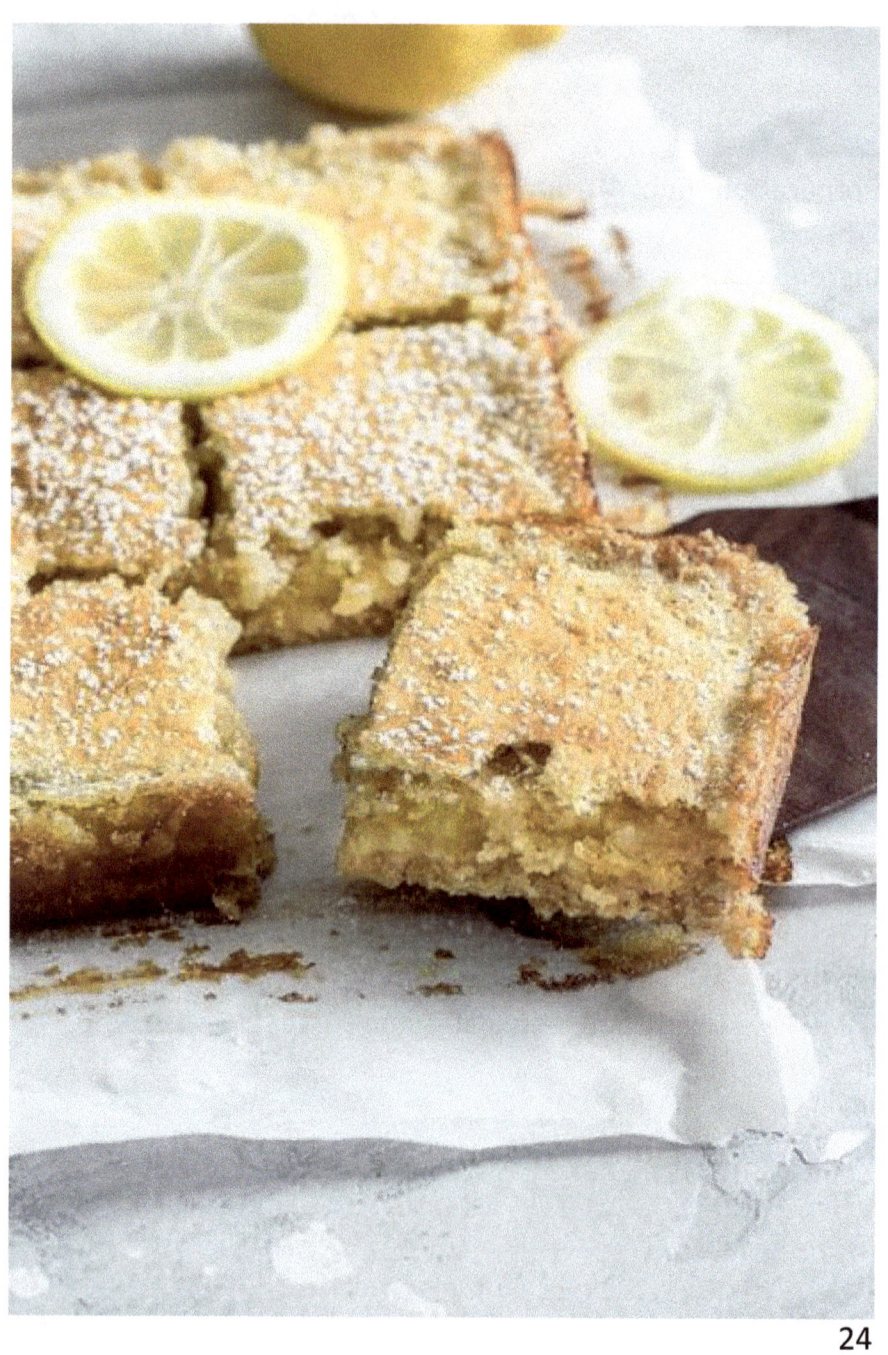

Chia Eggs and Lime

2 Servings

Preparation time: 30 minutes

Ingredients:

- 1 tablespoon lime juice
- ½ cup heavy cream
- 1 teaspoon sweet paprika
- Salt and black pepper to the taste
- 4 eggs, whisked
- 1 tablespoon chia seeds

Directions:

- In a sous vide bag, combine the eggs with the chia seeds and the other ingredients, toss, seal, introduce in your sous vide machine and cook in the water oven at 167 degrees F for 20 minutes.
- Divide the mix between plates and serve.

Broccoli Eggs

4 Servings

Preparation time: 40 minutes

Ingredients:

- Salt and black pepper to the taste
- 4 eggs, whisked
- 2 garlic cloves, minced
- 1 tablespoon chives, chopped
- ½ cup heavy cream
- 1 cup broccoli florets
- ½ teaspoon sweet paprika
- ½ teaspoon coriander, ground

Directions:

- In a sous vide bag, combine the eggs with the broccoli, paprika and the other ingredients, toss, seal, introduce in your sous vide machine and cook at 175 degrees F for 30 minutes.
- Divide everything between plates and serve for breakfast.

Ginger Tomatoes Eggs

4 Servings

Preparation time: 50 minutes

Ingredients:

- A drizzle of olive oil
- 1 red onion, chopped
- Salt and black pepper to the taste
- A pinch of red pepper, crushed
- 1 garlic clove, minced
- 1 tablespoon chives, chopped
- 1 cup cherry tomatoes, cubed
- 1 tablespoon ginger, grated
- 4 eggs, whisked

Directions:

- Heat up a pan with the oil over medium heat, add the ginger, onion and the other ingredients except the eggs, stir and cook for 10 minutes.

- In a bowl, combine the eggs with the ginger mix, stir, pour this into a sous vide bag, seal, submerge in the water oven and cook at 170 degrees F for 30 minutes.
- Divide everything between plates and serve for breakfast.

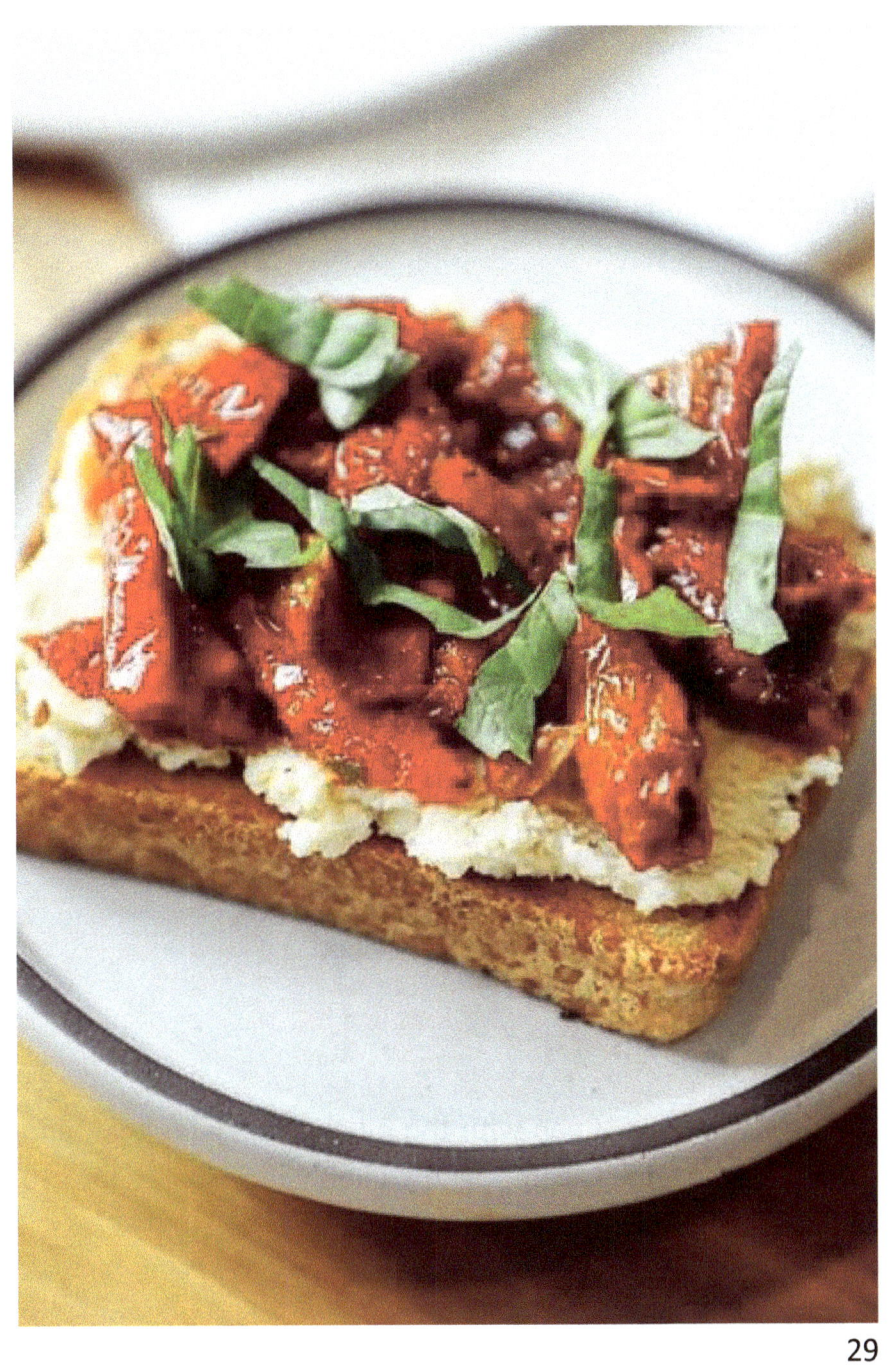

Bok Choy and Veggies Bowls

4 Servings

Preparation time: 40 minutes

Ingredients:

- 1 cup white mushrooms, halved
- 1 cup cherry tomatoes, halved
- 1 cup kalamata olives, pitted and halved
- Salt and black pepper to the taste
- ½ tablespoon red pepper flakes
- 1 red onion, chopped
- 1 bunch bok choy, chopped
- A drizzle of olive oil
- 2 tablespoons balsamic vinegar
- 2 tablespoons Worcestershire sauce
- 2 tablespoons chives, chopped

Directions:

- Heat up a pan with the oil over medium heat, add the mushrooms and onion and sauté for 10 minutes.

- In a sous vide bag, mix the bok choy with the tomatoes, mushroom mix and the remaining ingredients, seal, introduce in your sous vide machine and cook at 170 degrees F for 20 minutes.
- Divide the whole mix into bowls and serve for breakfast.

Bok Choy and Eggs

2 Servings

Preparation time: 30 minutes

Ingredients:

- ½ teaspoon chili powder
- 2 bunches bok choy, chopped
- 2 bacon slices, chopped
- Salt and black pepper to the taste
- A drizzle of avocado oil
- 2 garlic cloves, minced
- 4 eggs, whisked
- ½ teaspoon turmeric powder

Directions:

- In sous vide bag, combine the eggs with the bok choy and the other ingredients, toss, seal, submerge in the water bath and cook at 170 degrees F for 20 minutes.
- Divide between plates and serve for breakfast

Greens and Eggs

4 Servings

Preparation time: 30 minutes

Ingredients:

- 1 tablespoon lime juice
- 8 eggs, whisked
- ½ teaspoon chili powder
- Salt and black pepper to the taste
- 1 cup baby spinach
- 1 cup collard greens, chopped
- ¼ cup spring onions, chopped

Directions:

- In a sous vide bag, combine the greens with the eggs and the other ingredients, seal the bag, introduce in your sous vide machine and cook at 170 degrees F for 20 minutes.
- Divide between plates and serve for breakfast.

Eggs and Asparagus

4 Servings

Preparation time: 35 minutes

Ingredients:

- 4 eggs, whisked
- ½ teaspoon sweet paprika
- ½ teaspoon chili powder
- 1 cup cheddar cheese, grated
- ¼ cup red onion, chopped
- 1 pound asparagus spears, chopped
- Salt and black pepper to the taste

Directions:

- In a sous vide bag, combine the eggs with the eggs and the other ingredients, toss, seal, introduce in your sous vide machine and cook at 168 degrees F for 20 minutes.
- Divide between plates and serve for breakfast.

COCKTAILS AND INFUSIONS

Lavender Syrup

4 Servings

Preparation time: 1 hour 5 minutes

Ingredients:

- 1 cup water
- 1 cup sugar
- 1 tablespoon culinary grade dried lavender

Directions:

- Prepare your Sous Vide water bath using your immersion circulator and raise the temperature to 135-degrees Fahrenheit.
- Take a heavy-duty resealable zipper bag and add the water, lavender, and sugar.
- Seal it using the immersion method.
- Submerge it underwater and cook for about 1 hour.
- Once done, let it cool down to room temperature and strain through a metal mesh.
- Serve chilled!

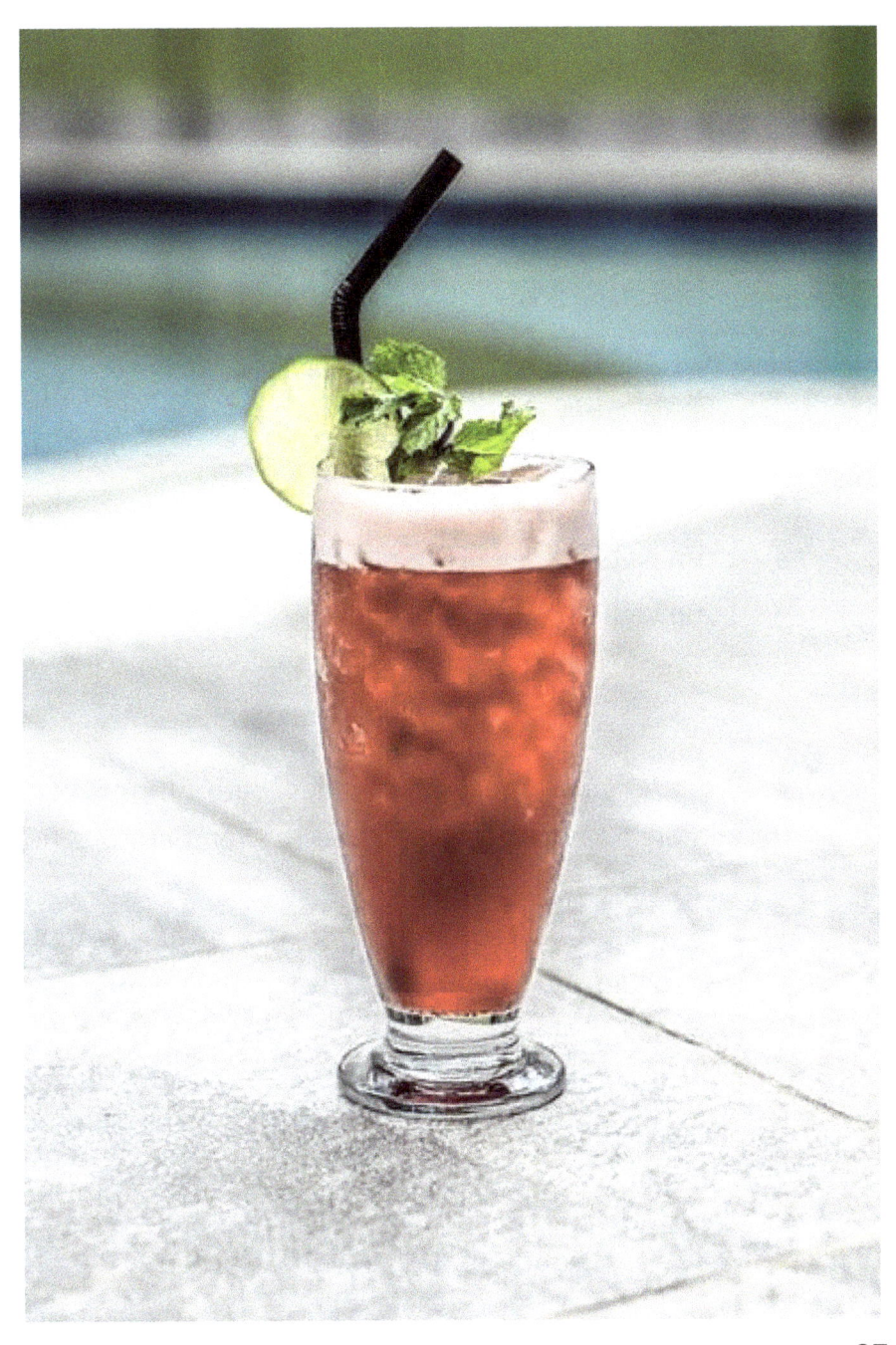

Thyme Liqueur

12 Servings

Preparation time: 1 hour 35 minutes

Ingredients:

- Zest of 8 large oranges
- 4 sprigs fresh thyme
- 1 cup ultrafine sugar
- 1 cup water
- 1 cup vodka

Directions:

- Prepare your Sous Vide water bath using your immersion circulator and raise the temperature to 180-degrees Fahrenheit.
- Add all the listed ingredients to a heavy-duty resealable zip bag and seal using the immersion method.
- Cook for 90 minutes.
- Strain the mixture and serve chilled!

Vodka Lemon Meyer

6 Servings

Preparation time: 1 hour 35 minutes

Ingredients:

- 1 cup vodka
- 1 cup granulated sugar
- 1 cup freshly squeezed Meyer lemon
- Zest of 3 Meyer lemons

Directions:

- Prepare your Sous Vide water bath using your immersion circulator and raise the temperature to 135-degrees Fahrenheit.
- Take a resealable zip bag and add all the listed ingredients.
- Seal the bag using the immersion method. Submerge and cook for about 2 hours.
- Once done, strain the mixture through a fine metal mesh strainer into a medium bowl.
- Chill the mixture overnight and serve!

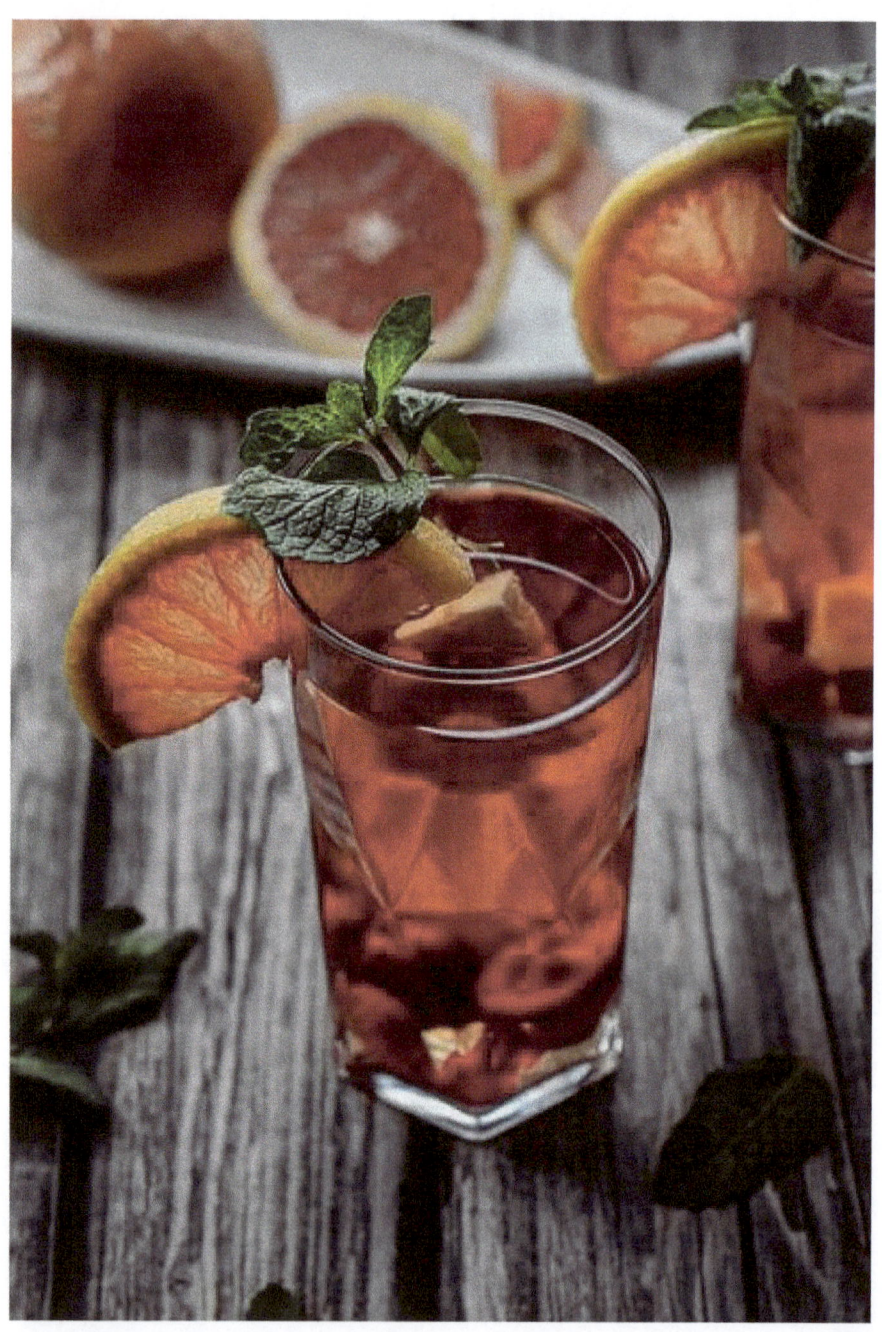

Rosemary & Lemon Vodka

5 Servings

Preparation time: 1 hour 35 minutes

Ingredients:

- 1 bottle vodka
- Zest of 6 large lemons
- 5 sprigs fresh rosemary

Directions:

- Prepare your Sous Vide water bath using your immersion circulator and raise the temperature to 145-degrees Fahrenheit.
- Take a heavy-duty resealable zip bag and add all the listed ingredients.
- Seal using the immersion method and cook for 3 hours.
- Once done, transfer the contents through a strainer and allow it to cool.
- Serve!

Bloody Mary Vodka

20 Servings

Preparation time: 1 hour 35 minutes

Ingredients:

- 1 bottle vodka
- 6 quartered roma tomatoes
- 1 Anaheim pepper, stemmed and seeds removed, sliced into ½ inch pieces
- ¼ onion, peeled and sliced into ½-inch pieces
- 6 whole garlic cloves, peeled
- 1 thinly sliced jalapeno pepper
- 1 tablespoon whole black peppercorns
- Zest of 3 large limes

Directions:

- Prepare your Sous Vide water bath using your immersion circulator and raise the temperature to 145-degrees Fahrenheit.

- Add all the listed ingredients to your resealable zipper bag.
- Seal using the immersion method.
- Cook for about 3 hours and transfer the contents through a mesh strainer.
- Serve!

Coffee Liquor

20 Servings

Preparation time: 1 hour 35 minutes

Ingredients:

- 1 bottle vodka
- 32 oz. strong black coffee
- 2 cups granulated sugar
- ½ cup coffee beans
- 2 split vanilla beans

Directions:

- Prepare your Sous Vide water bath using your immersion circulator and raise the temperature to 145-degrees Fahrenheit.
- Take a heavy-duty large resealable zip bag and add all the listed ingredients.
- Seal the bag using the immersion method.
- Cook for about 3 hours underwater.
- Once done, transfer the contents through a fine mesh strainer and let it cool.
- Serve!

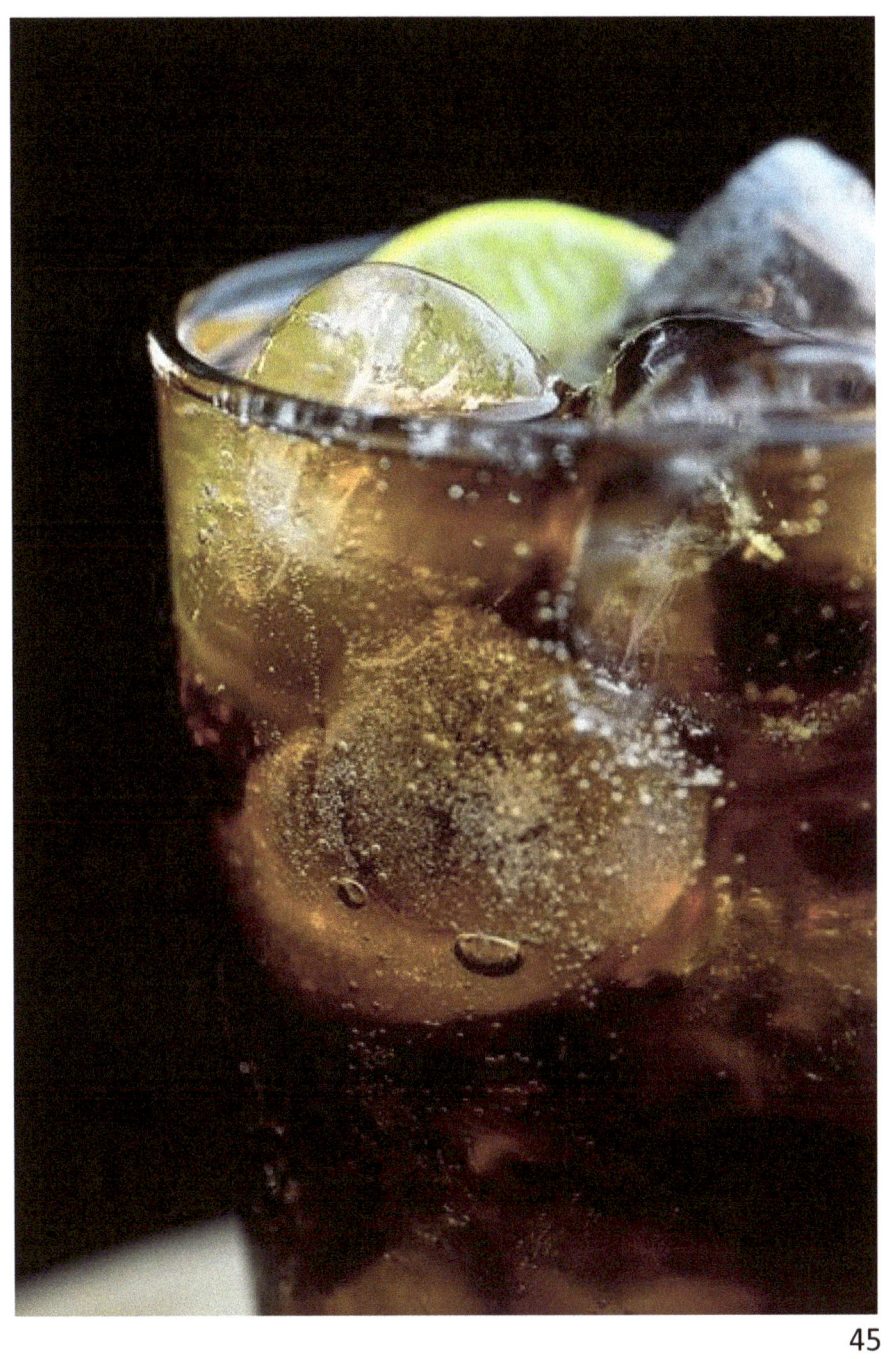

Honey Ginger Shrub

6 Servings

Preparation time: 1 hour 35 minutes

Ingredients

- 1 cup water
- ½ cup honey
- ½ cup balsamic vinegar
- 1 tablespoon freshly grated ginger
- Bourbon whiskey
- Club soda
- Lemon wedges as required

Directions:

- Prepare your Sous Vide water bath using your immersion circulator and raise the temperature to 134-degrees Fahrenheit.
- Take a resealable zipper bag and add the water, vinegar, honey, ginger, and seal it using the immersion method.
- Submerge and cook for about 2 hours.

- Once cooked, strain the mixture through a fine metal mesh strainer into a medium bowl.
- Chill the mixture overnight.
- Serve with one-part whiskey and one-part club soda in a glass over ice.
- Garnish with a lemon wedge and serve!

Cherry Bourbon

8 Servings

Preparation time: 1 hour 35 minutes

Ingredients

- 1 lb. fresh cherries
- 1½ cups bourbon

Directions:

- Prepare your Sous Vide water bath using your immersion circulator and raise the temperature to 135-degrees Fahrenheit.
- Then, pit the cherries using a cherry pitter. (if using)
- Add the cherries and bourbon to a resealable zipper bag.
- Seal using the immersion method and mash the cherries. Cook for 2 hours.
- Let the mixture cool and strain it to a bowl through a fine metal mesh
- Pour in the bottles and serve chilled!

Bacon Vodka

10 Servings

Preparation time: 1 hour 20 minutes

Ingredients:

- 2 cups vodka
- 8 oz. bacon
- 3 tablespoons reserved bacon grease

Directions:

- Prepare your Sous Vide water bath using your immersion circulator and raise the temperature to 150-degrees Fahrenheit.
- Bake the bacon for 16 minutes at 400-degrees Fahrenheit.
- Allow the mixture to cool.
- Add all the ingredients to a resealable bag and seal using the immersion method.
- Cook for 45 minutes.
- Strain the liquid into a bowl and chill until a fat layer forms.
- Remove and skim off the fat layer, strain using cheesecloth once again.
- Serve chilled!

LUNCH

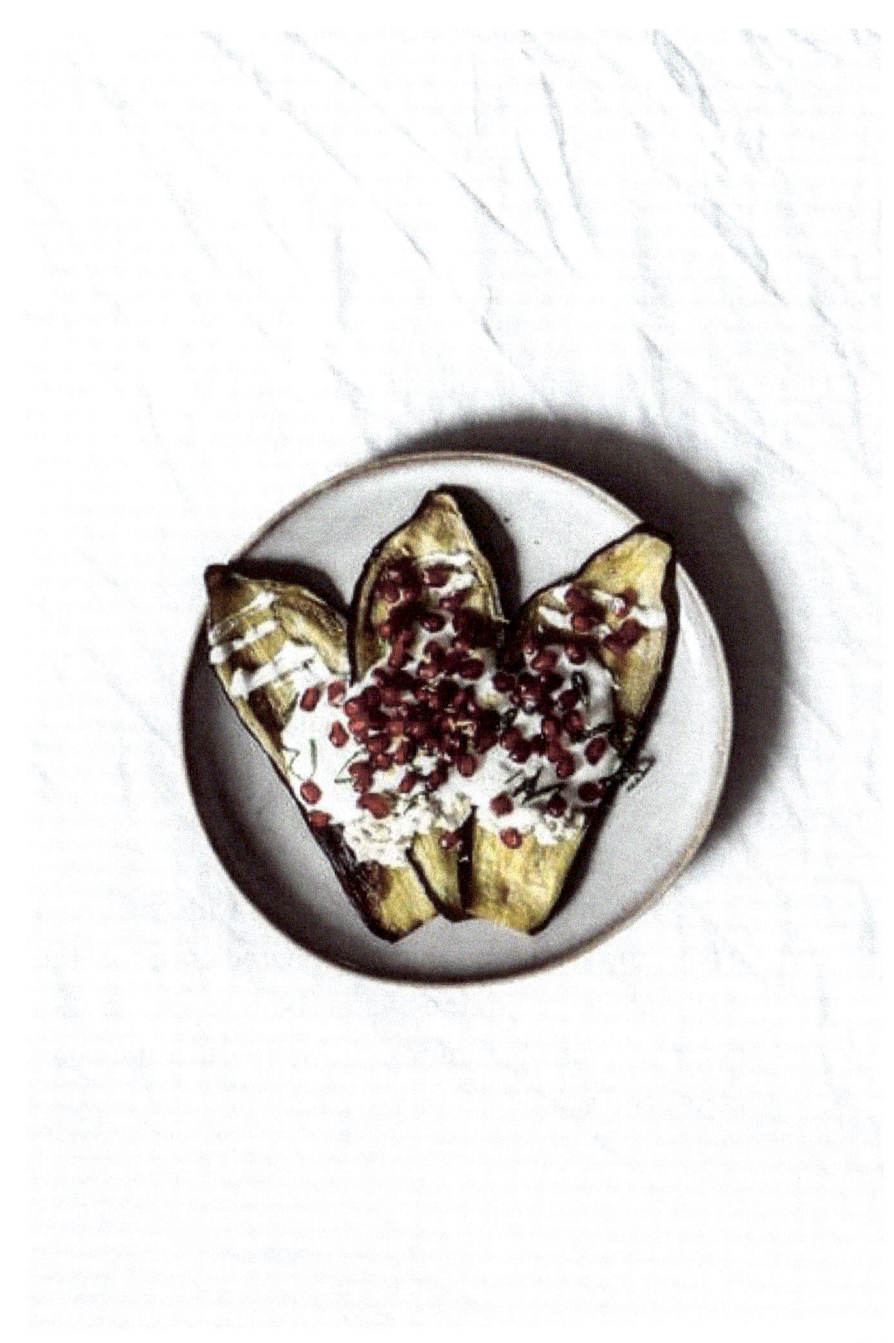

Peppers and Green Beans

4 Servings

Preparation time: 50 minutes

Ingredients:

- 2 red bell peppers, cut into wedges
- 1 pound green beans, trimmed and halved
- 2 tablespoons soy sauce
- Juice of ½ lime
- A pinch of salt and black pepper
- 2 garlic cloves, minced
- 1 cup black olives, pitted and halved

Directions:

- In a sous vide bag, mix the peppers with the green beans, soy sauce and the other ingredients, seal the bag, submerge in the water bath, cook at 180 degrees F for 35 minutes, divide the mix between plates and serve.

Savory Oatmeal with Mushrooms

4 Servings

Preparation Time: 8 hours 10 minutes

Ingredients:

- 1 cup steel-cut oats
- 4 cups water
- 1/2 teaspoon sea salt
- 1/2 teaspoon ground black pepper
- 1/2 teaspoon cayenne pepper
- 2 tablespoons grapeseed oil
- 8 ounces brown mushrooms, sliced
- 1/2 medium onion, chopped
- 4 cloves garlic, minced
- 3 sprigs fresh thyme
- 1 cup baby spinach

Directions:

- Preheat a sous vide water bath to 175 degrees F.
- Place steel-cut oats, water, salt, black pepper, and cayenne pepper in cooking pouches; seal tightly.

- Submerge the cooking pouches in the water bath; cook for 4 hours; reserve.
- Heat the oil in a pan that is preheated over a moderately high heat. Sauté the mushrooms, onion, and garlic until softened.
- Now, add fresh thyme and continue cooking an additional 5 minutes. Spoon mushroom mixture over the prepared oatmeal. Top with baby spinach and serve warm. Bon appétit!

Spicy Kidney Beans

3 Servings

Preparation Time: 9 hours 35 minutes

Ingredients:

- 2 cups dried red kidney beans
- 3 cloves garlic, crushed
- 2 bay leaves
- 1/2 teaspoon black peppercorns
- 1 teaspoon cayenne pepper
- Sea salt, to taste
- 5 cups water
- 2 tablespoons olive oil
- 1 yellow onion, peeled and chopped
- 2 celery stalks, finely diced
- 2 bell peppers, finely diced
- 1/2 teaspoon chili flakes

Directions:

- Preheat a sous vide water bath to 194 degrees F.

- Place red kidney beans, garlic, bay leaves, black peppercorns, cayenne pepper, salt, and water in cooking pouches; seal tightly.
- Submerge the cooking pouches in the water bath; cook for 6 hours 30 minutes. Remove the beans form the cooking pouches, reserving the cooking liquid.
- Heat olive oil in a pan that is preheated over a moderate heat. Once hot, sauté the onions, celery and peppers until they are softened.
- Add the cooking liquid to deglaze the bottom of your pan. Add reserved beans and chili flakes and cook an additional 5 minutes or until heated through. Bon appétit!

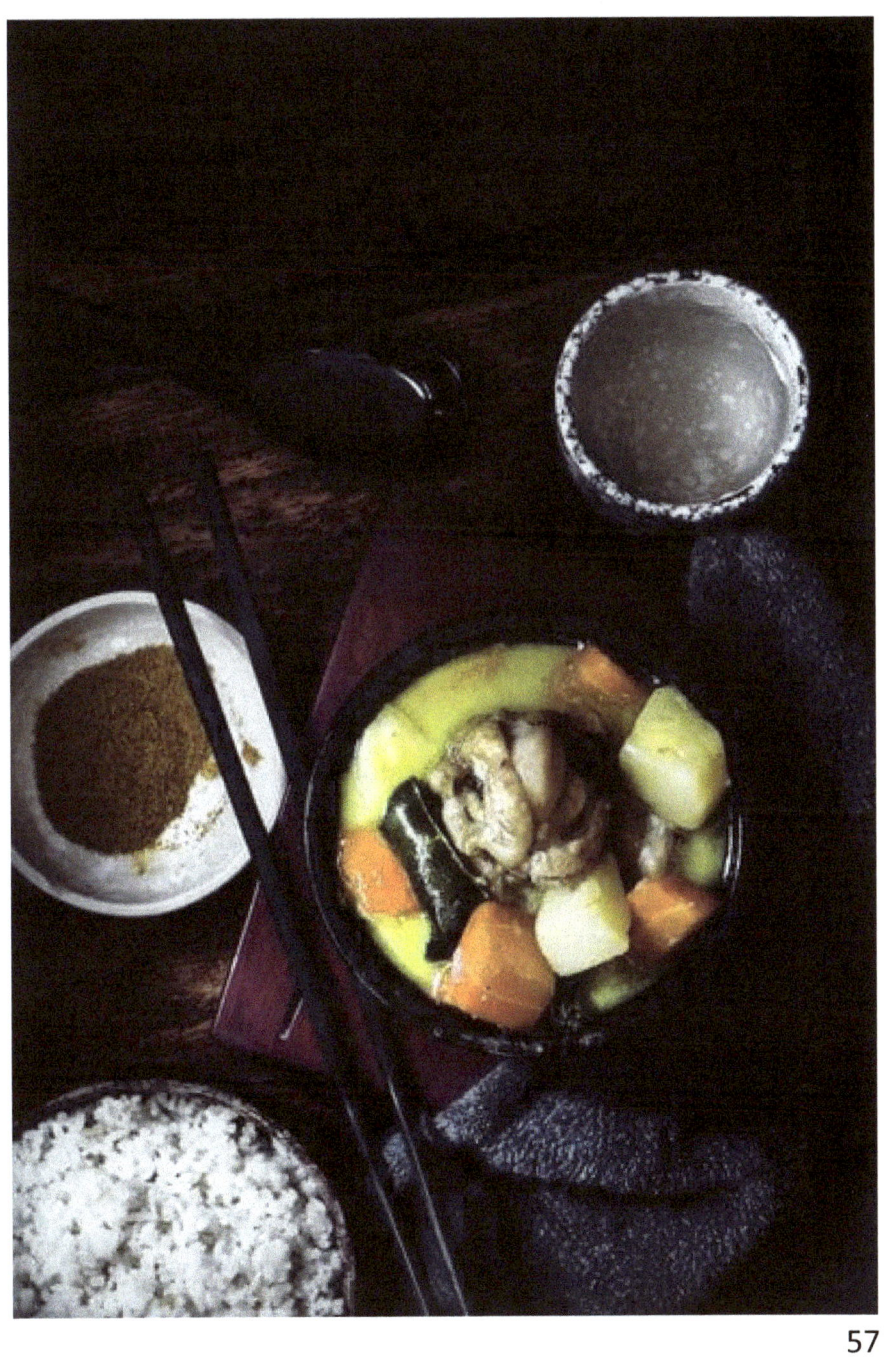

Delicious Lentil Curry

4 Servings

Preparation Time: 4 hours 40 minutes

Ingredients:

- 2 tablespoons grape seed oil
- 1 cup leeks, chopped
- 2 parsnips, chopped
- 2 carrots, chopped
- 2 stalks celery, chopped
- 2 cloves garlic, crushed
- Sea salt, to taste
- 1/3 teaspoon freshly ground black pepper
- 3 cups water
- 2 cups yellow lentils
- 2 sprigs fresh rosemary
- 2 sprigs fresh thyme
- 2 bay leaves
- 1 tablespoon curry powder
- 1 teaspoon garam masala
- 1/2 teaspoon fresh ginger, ground
- 1 cup full-fat coconut milk

Directions:

- Preheat a sous vide water bath to 183 degrees F.
- Heat the oil in a pan over moderate heat. Once hot, sauté the leeks, parsnip, carrots, celery, and garlic for 4 minutes.
- Add the salt and black pepper. Place this sautéed mixture in cooking pouches; add the water, lentils, rosemary, thyme, and bay leaves to the pouches; seal tightly.
- Submerge the cooking pouches in the water bath; cook for 1 hour 30 minutes.
- Transfer the contents of the cooking pouches to a large stockpot; add the remaining ingredients and let it simmer an additional 10 minutes or until thoroughly heated.
- Ladle into individual bowls and serve warm.

Fried Tofu in Peanut Sauce

3 Servings

Preparation Time: 4 hours 40 minutes

Ingredients:

- 16 ounces firm tofu, drained and sliced
- 1 tablespoon peanut oil
- 2 cloves garlic, roughly minced
- Celery salt and freshly ground black pepper, to taste
- 1 teaspoon curry powder
- Peanut Sauce:
- 2 tablespoons peanut butter
- 4 tablespoons soymilk
- 1 tablespoon soy sauce
- 1/2 teaspoon chili powder
- 1/2 teaspoon mustard seeds
- 1/2 teaspoon celery seeds
- Salt, to taste

Directions:

- Preheat a Sous vide water bath to 183 degrees F.

- Add tofu, 1 tablespoon of peanut oil, garlic, salt, black pepper, and curry powder to cooking pouches; seal tightly.
- Submerge the cooking pouches in the water bath; cook for 1 hour 30 minutes; reserve cooking liquids.
- Heat a cast-iron pan over moderately high heat; fry tofu slices for 3 to 4 minutes or until they are lightly browned on both sides.
- In a saucepan, simmer peanut butter, soymilk, soy sauce, chili powder, mustard seeds, and celery seeds for 2 to 3 minutes.
- Add the reserved tofu and sprinkle with salt to taste. Serve warm. Bon appétit!

Grand Marnier

12 Servings

Preparation Time: 1 hour 35 minutes

Ingredients:

- Zest, 8 large orange
- 2 cups brandy
- ½ cup ultrafine sugar

Directions:

- Prepare your Sous Vide water bath using your immersion circulator and raise the temperature to 180ºF.
- Add all the listed ingredients to a resealable zip bag.
- Seal using the immersion method.
- Cook for 90 minutes.
- Strain and discard the orange zest.
- Allow it to chill and serve when needed!

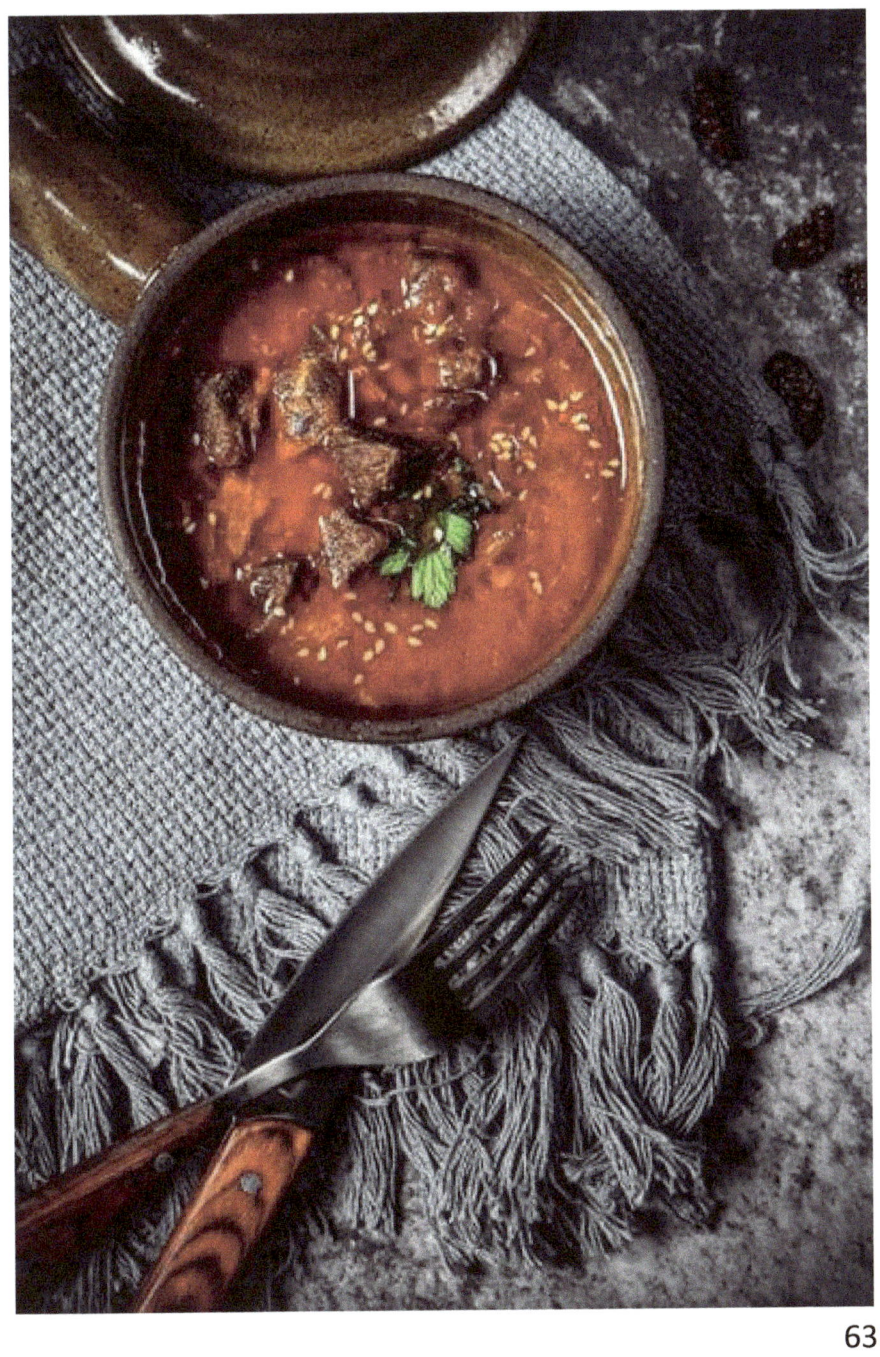

Red Wine Plum Shrub

8 Servings

Preparation Time: 1 hour 35 minutes

Ingredients:

- 2 cups red plum, pitted, diced
- 1 cup ultrafine sugar
- 1 cup red wine
- 1 cup red wine vinegar
- 1 cinnamon stick
- 1 clove
- ½ teaspoon vanilla bean paste

Directions:

- Prepare your Sous Vide water bath using your immersion circulator and raise the temperature to 180ºF.
- Add all the listed ingredients to a resealable bag.
- Seal using the immersion method and cook for 90 minutes.
- Strain and discard the cinnamon stick, clove, and plums.
- Chill and serve!

Lamb Shoulder

10 Servings

Preparation Time: 8 hours

Ingredients:

- 2 pounds lamb shoulder, bones removed
- 1 garlic clove
- 2 tbsps olive oil
- 2 rosemary sprigs
- Salt and pepper to taste

Directions:

- Preheat the water bath to 180ºF.
- Season the lamb shank with salt and pepper.
- Put the lamb into the vacuum bag, adding rosemary sprigs, olive oil and garlic.
- Seal the bag.
- Set the cooking timer for 8 hours.
- Serve with boiled potatoes pouring the cooking juices over.

SNACKS

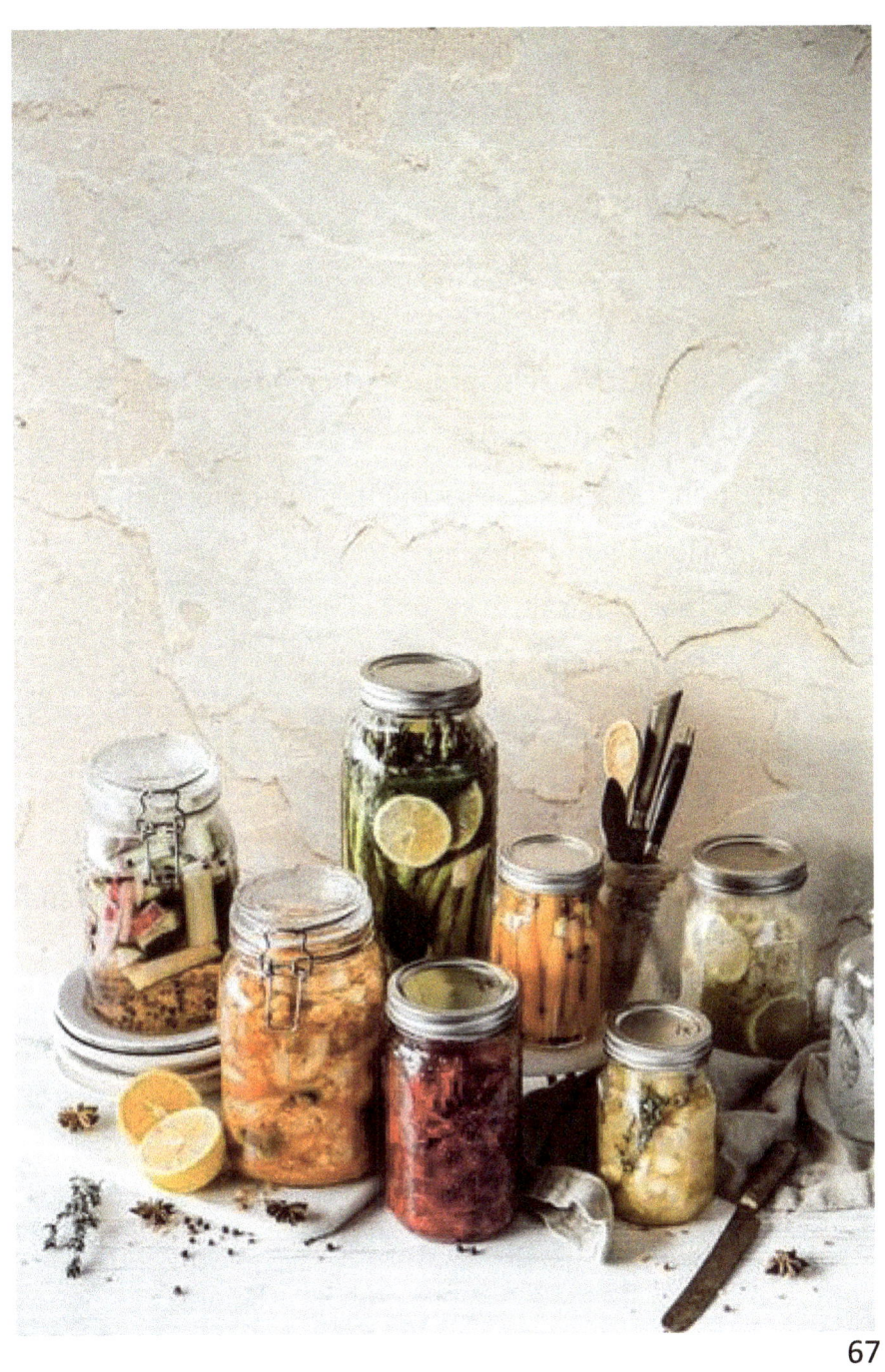

Bacon Brussels sprouts

4 Servings

Preparation time: 1 hour 20 minutes

Ingredients:

- 1 pound Brussels sprouts, trimmed and halved
- 2 tablespoons butter
- 2 ounces thick-cut bacon, fried and chopped
- 2 cloves garlic, minced
- ¼ teaspoon salt
- ¼ teaspoon pepper

Directions:

- Preheat the water bath to 183°F
- Combine Brussels sprouts, butter, garlic, salt, and pepper in a bag. Seal and place in water bath.
- Cook 1 hour. Meanwhile, preheat oven to 400°F
- After 1 hour has passed, spread Brussels sprouts on a cookie sheet. Bake for 5 minutes or until edges of sprouts are crisp and lightly browned.

Okra with Chili Yogurt

5 Servings

Preparation time: 1 hour 15 minutes

Ingredients:

- 5 lbs fresh okra
- 4 tablespoons olive oil
- 1 ½ tablespoons lime zest
- 2 cloves garlic, crushed
- Salt and white pepper, to taste
- Yogurt:
- 1 cup Greek yogurt
- 2 teaspoons chili powder
- ¼ cup chopped cilantro

Directions:

- Preheat your Sous Vide to 178F.
- Divide the fresh okra among two cooking bags.
- Drizzle the okra with 2 ½ tablespoons olive oil (divided per bag, lime zest, and season to taste. Add one clove garlic per pouch.
- Vacuum seal the bags and submerge in water.

- Cook the okra 1 hour. Remove from a water bath and drain the accumulated liquid in a bowl. Place the okra in a separate bowl.
- In a medium bowl, combine Greek yogurt, chili powder, cilantro, and accumulated okra water. Stir to combine.
- Heat remaining olive oil in a skillet over medium-high heat.
- Fry okra in the heated oil for 2 minutes.
- Serve warm with chili yogurt.

Sous Vide Ratatouille

4 Servings

Preparation time: 40 minutes

Ingredients:

- 2 red bell peppers, seeded and sliced
- 2 yellow bell peppers, seeded and sliced
- 2 green bell peppers, seeded and sliced
- 4 small green zucchinis, sliced
- 4 yellow zucchinis, sliced
- 4 shallots, sliced
- 4 cloves garlic
- 10 brown mushrooms
- 6 small tomatoes, sliced
- 2 tablespoons soy sauce
- 4 tablespoons chopped mixed herbs (parsley, coriander, mint)
- 2 pinches sugar
- 2 pinches black pepper
- ½ cup olive oil
- Salt, to taste

Directions:

- Before you start, cut the vegetables into equal-size pieces. This way you will ensure all ingredients are cooked at the same time.
- Preheat your Sous Vide to 150F.
- Combine all ingredients in a large bowl. Toss gently to coat with oil.
- Divide the veggies between four cooking bags.
- Vacuum seal the bags and submerge under heated water.
- Cook the vegetables for 30 minutes.
- Heat some oil in a wok pan.
- Add the veggies and stir-fry for 30 seconds.
- Serve warm.

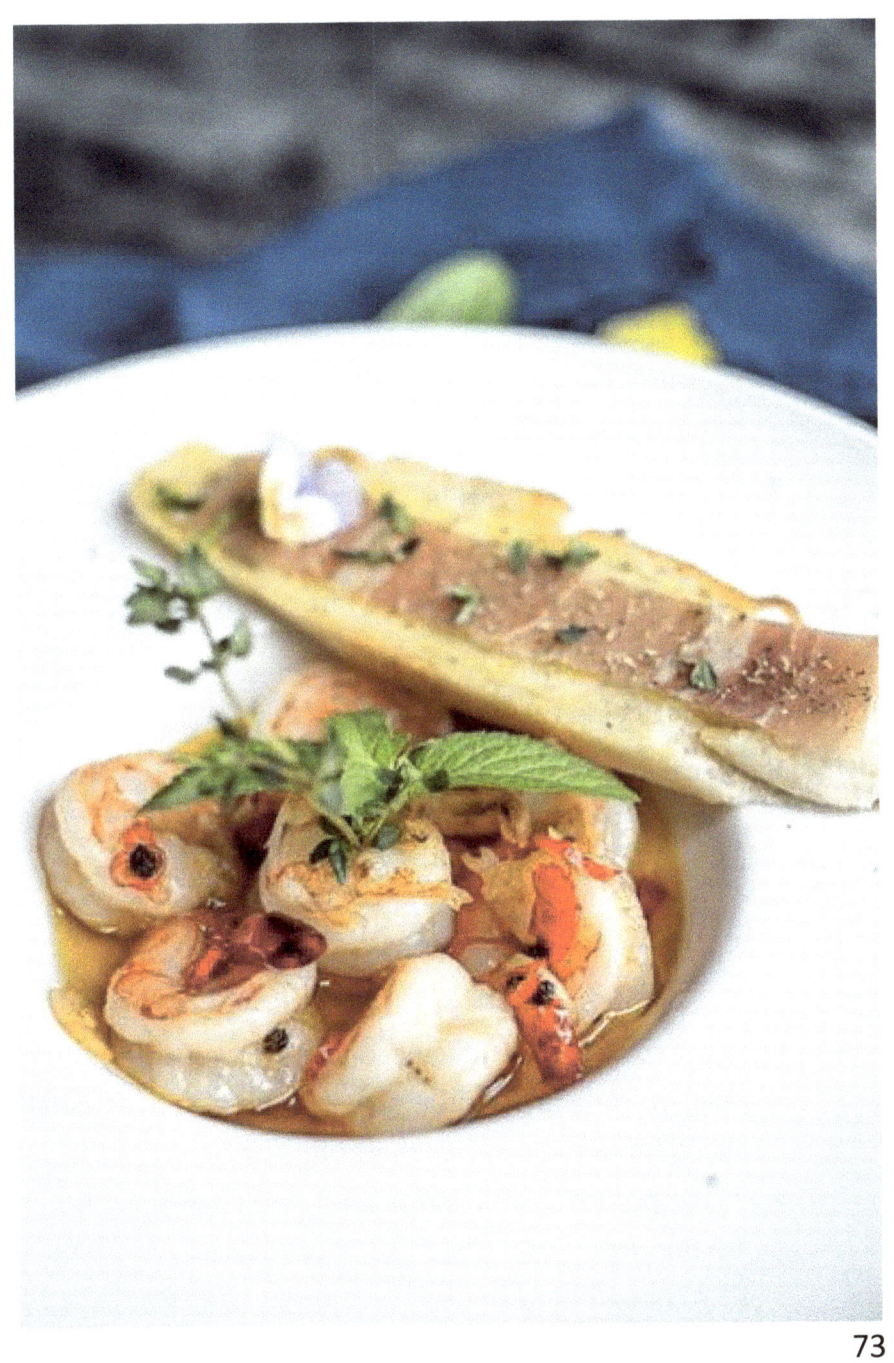

Potato Salad

6 Servings

Preparation time: 1 hour 10 minutes

Ingredients:

- 1 ½ pounds yellow potatoes or red potatoes (waxy potatoes work best
- ½ cup chicken stock
- Salt and pepper to taste
- 4 oz. thick cut bacon, sliced into about ¼-inch slices
- ½ cup chopped onion
- 1/3 cup cider vinegar
- 4 scallions, thinly sliced

Directions:

- Set Sous Vide cooker to 185F.
- Cut potatoes into ¾-inch thick cubes.
- Place potatoes and chicken stock to the zip-lock bag, making sure they are in a single layer; seal using immersion water method.
- Place potatoes in a water bath and cook for 1 hour 30 minutes.

- Meanwhile, in the last 15 minutes, heat non-stick skillet over medium-high heat. Add bacon and cook until crisp; remove bacon and add chopped onions. Cook until soften for 5-7 minutes.
- Add vinegar and cook until reduced slightly.
- Remove potatoes from the water bath and place them in skillet, with the cooking water.
- Continue cooking for few minutes until liquid thickens.
- Remove potatoes from the heat and stir in scallions; toss to combine.
- Serve while still hot.

Rosemary Fava Beans

4 Servings

Preparation time: 80 minutes

Ingredients:

- 25 lbs fava beans, cleaned
- ½ teaspoon salt
- 2 sprigs rosemary
- ¼ teaspoon caraway seeds
- 1 pinch black pepper
- 3 tablespoons cold butter

Directions:

- Preheat your Sous Vide to 176F.
- Blanche the fava beans in simmering water 1 minute. Drain and divide between two Sous Vide bags.
- Season the beans with salt, pepper, and caraway seeds.

- Add 1 tablespoon butter per bag, and vacuum seals the bags.
- Submerge the bags in water and cook for 70 minutes.
- Remove the veggies from the bag.
- Heat remaining butter in a skillet. Toss in the beans and coat the beans with butter.
- Serve warm.

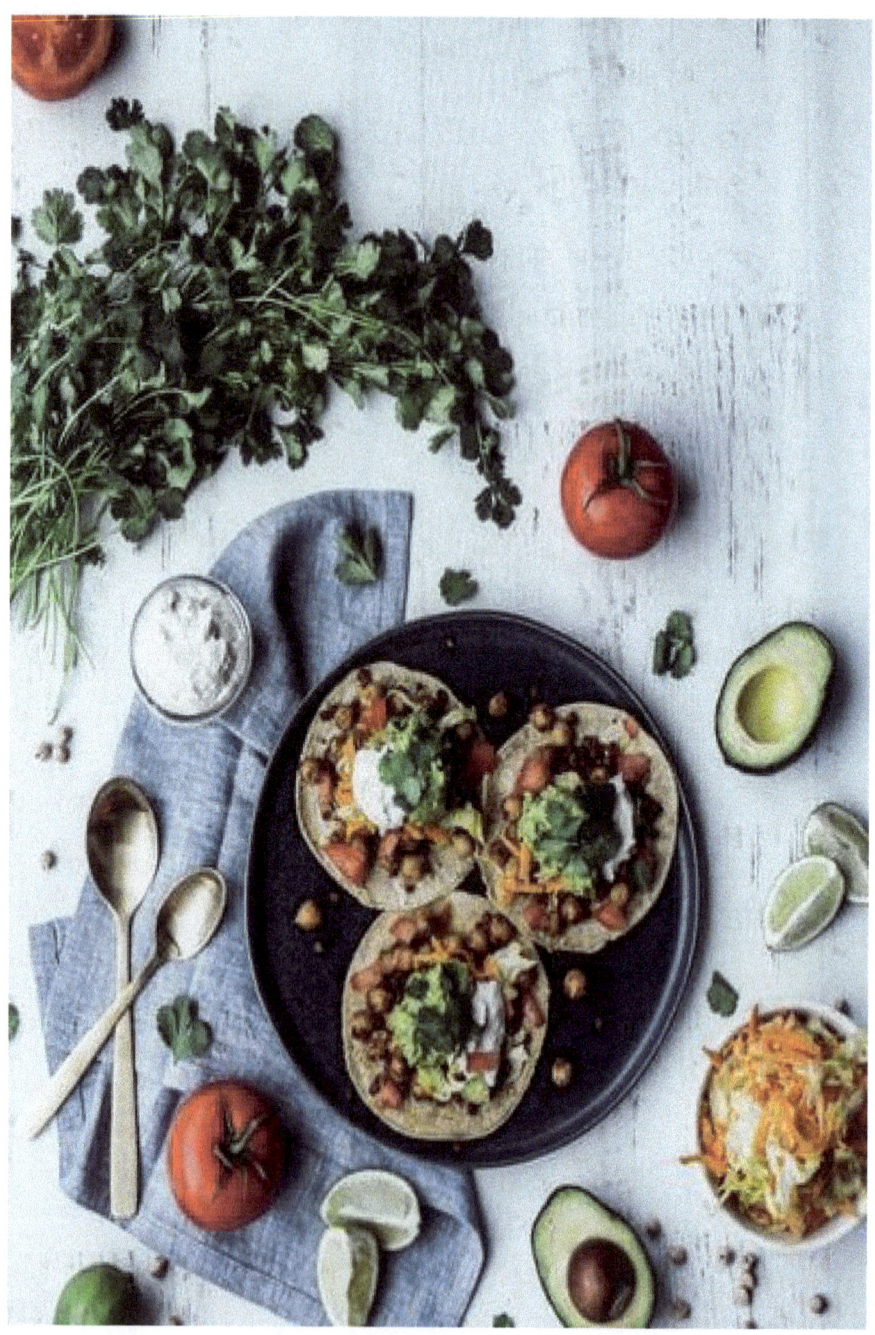

Thyme Lard Broad Beans

4 Servings

Preparation time: 1 hour 10 minutes

Ingredients:

- 5 lbs broad beans
- 4 sprigs thyme
- 3oz. lard
- 1 pinch red pepper flakes

Directions:

- Preheat Sous Vide cooker to 176F.
- Trim the beans and blanch in simmering water for 30 seconds. Rinse the beans under cold water.
- Divide the beans between two bags. Add two sprigs thyme per bag.
- Chop the lard and sprinkle over the beans, along with red pepper flakes.
- Vacuum seal the bag and submerge in a water bath.
- Cook the beans 60 minutes.

Finishing steps:

- Remove the beans from Sous Vide cooker and submerge in ice-cold water for 2-3 minutes.
- Open the bags and serve the beans.

Tomato Confit

4 Servings

Preparation time: 45 minutes

Ingredients:

- 25 lbs cherry tomatoes (red, orange, yellow
- 1 pinch Fleur de sel
- 6 black peppercorns
- 1 teaspoon cane sugar
- 2 tablespoons Bianco Aceto Balsamico
- 2 sprigs rosemary

Directions:

- Preheat Sous Vide to 126F.
- Heat water in a pot and bring to simmer.
- Make a small incision at the bottom of each tomato.
- Place the tomatoes into simmering water and simmer for 30 seconds.
- Remove from the water and peel their skin.
- Divide the tomatoes between two Souse Vide bags.

- Sprinkle the tomatoes with salt, peppercorns, sugar, and Aceto Balsamico. Add 1 sprig rosemary per bag.
- Vacuum-seal the bags, but just to 90%. Tomatoes are soft, and they can turn into mush.
- Submerge tomatoes in water and cook 20 minutes.

Finishing steps:

- Remove the tomatoes from Sous Vide cooker and submerge in ice-cold water for 5 minutes.
- Transfer the tomatoes to a bowl, and serve with fresh mozzarella.

Pears in Pomegranate Juice

8 Servings

Preparation time: 50 minutes

Ingredients:

- 8 pears
- 5 cups pomegranate juice
- ¾ cup sugar
- 1 cinnamon stick
- ¼ teaspoon nutmeg
- ¼ teaspoon ground cloves
- ¼ teaspoon allspice

Directions:

- Preheat Sous Vide cooker to 176F.
- Combine all ingredients, except the pears.
- Simmer until the liquid is reduced by half.
- Strain and place aside.
- Gently scrub the pears or peel if desired.
- Place each pear is sous Vide bag, and pour in some poaching liquid. Make sure each pear has the same level of poaching liquid.
- Vacuum seal the pears and submerge in water.

- Cook 30 minutes.
- Open bags and remove pears carefully. Slice the pears and place onto a plate.
- Cook the juices in a saucepan until thick.
- Drizzle over pears.
- Serve warm.

DINNER

Crab Zucchini Roulade with Mousse

4 Servings

Preparation Time: 40 minutes + inactive time

Ingredients:

- 3 lbs crab legs and claws
- 2 tablespoons olive oil
- 1 medium zucchini
- Salt and pepper, to taste

Mousse:

- 1 avocado, peeled, pitted
- 1 tablespoon Worcestershire sauce
- 2 tablespoons crème Fraiche
- 2 tablespoons fresh lime juice
- Salt, to taste

Directions:

- Preheat Sous vide cooker to 185F.
- Place the claws and legs in a Sous Vide bag and vacuum seal.

- Submerge the bag with content in a water bath. Cook the crab 10 minutes.

Finishing steps:

- Slice the zucchini with a vegetable peeler. This way you will have some skinny strips.
- Remove the crab from the water bath and crack the shell.
- Flake the meat and transfer into a bowl. Add olive oil, salt, and pepper, and stir to bind gently.
- Make the mousse; in a food blender, blend the avocado and crème Fraiche until smooth.
- Stir in the remaining ingredients and spoon the mixture into piping bag.
- Arrange the zucchini slices on aluminum foil and fill with the crab meat.
- Roll up the zucchinis and crab into a log and refrigerate 30 minutes.
- To serve; cut the roulade into four pieces. Serve onto a plate with some avocado mousse.
- Enjoy.

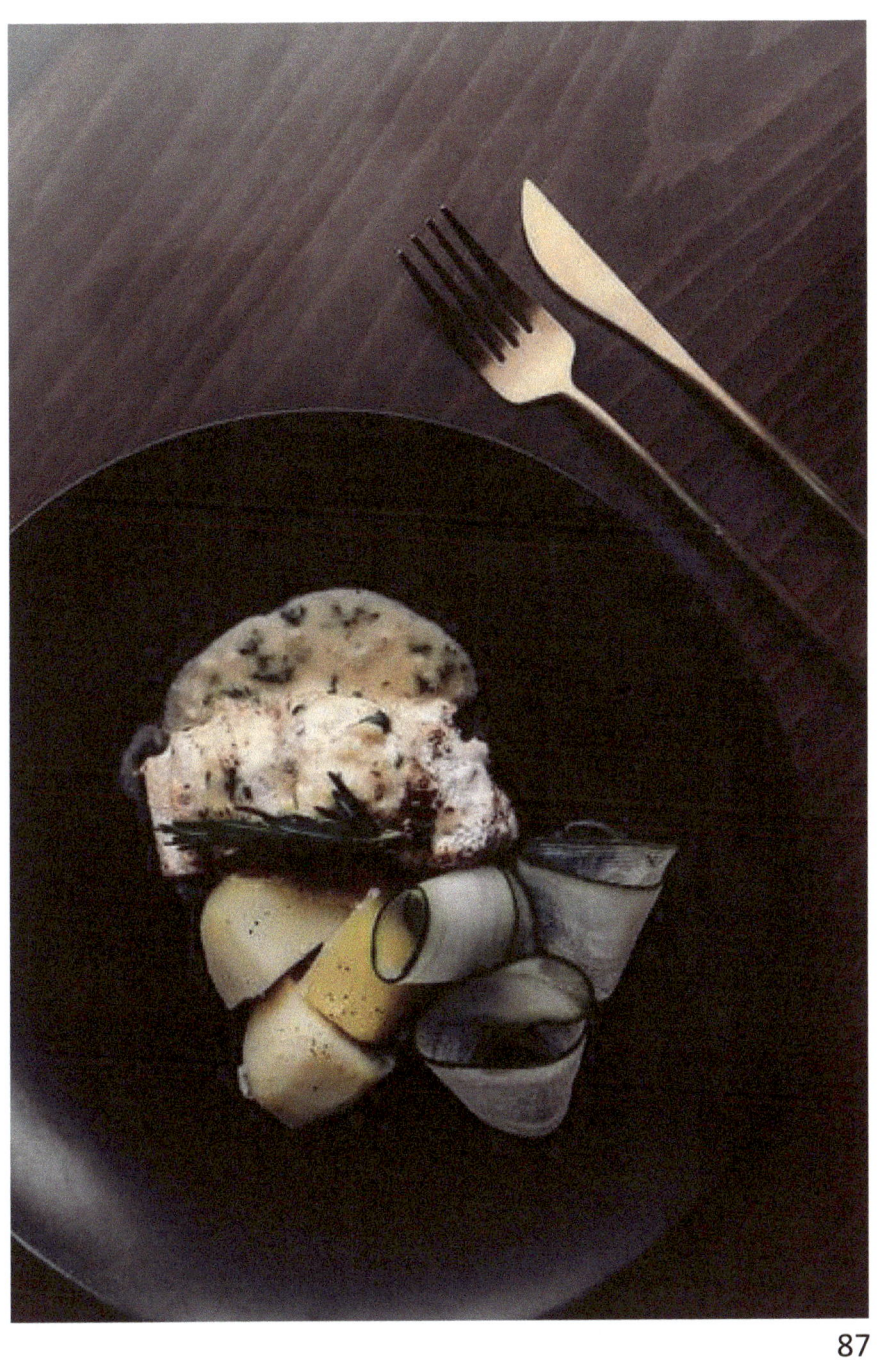

Herbed Prawns

4 Servings

Preparation Time: 50 minutes

Ingredients:

Prawns:

- 12 large prawns, cleaned
- 3 tablespoons olive oil
- 1 cup basil, chopped
- ½ cup parsley, chopped
- ½ cup dill, chopped
- 1 large organic lemon, sliced
- 2 chili peppers, seeded, chopped

Pasta:

- 1 cup pine nuts
- ¾ cup basil
- ¾ cup parsley
- ¼ cup dill
- ½ cup olive oil
- 2 cloves garlic

- Salt and pepper, to taste
- 1lb. spaghetti, cooked

Directions:

- Preheat Sous Vide cooker to 134F.
- In a bowl, combine all ingredients. Toss to coat the prawns with olive oil and herbs.
- Transfer the coated prawns into Sous Vide cooking bag, and top with lemon slices. Vacuum seal the bag.
- Submerge the prawns in the water bath and cook the prawns for 25 minutes.

Finishing steps:

- While the prawns are cooking, make the pesto. In a food blender, blend pine nuts, basil, parsley, dill, and garlic until just smooth. Set the blender to run on low and stream in the oil. Mix 2 minutes.
- Toss the spaghetti with pesto.
- Open the bag and spread the prawns over the spaghetti.
- Serve.

Elk Steak

4 Servings

Preparation Time: 2 hours 10 minutes

Ingredients:

For Steaks:

- 4 elk steaks
- sea salt, to taste
- bacon Fat, as required

For Brussels Sprouts:

- 3-4 cups brussels sprouts, trimmed
- 1-2 tablespoons coconut oil
- sea salt, to taste
- 1-2 tablespoons balsamic vinegar

Directions:

- Attach the sous vide immersion circulator using an adjustable clamp to a Cambro container or pot filled with water and preheat to 130°F.
- Season steaks evenly with salt.

- Into a cooking pouch, add the steaks. Seal pouch tightly after squeezing out the excess air. Place pouch in sous vide bath and set the cooking time for 1-2 hours.
- Preheat the oven to 400°F.
- For the Brussels sprouts: In a pan of boiling water, cook Brussels sprouts for 3 minutes.
- Drain well and immediately plunge into a large bowl of ice water to cool.
- After cooling, cut Brussels sprouts in half.
- Arrange Brussels sprout onto a baking sheet. Top with some coconut oil and sprinkle with salt.
- Place baking sheet in oven and bake for 2 minutes.
- Remove baking sheet from oven and toss sprouts well.
- Bake for a further 20 minutes, tossing once midway.
- Remove sprouts from oven and transfer into a bowl with the vinegar, and toss to coat.
- Remove steak pouch from sous vide bath and carefully open it. Remove steaks from pouch. With paper towels, pat steaks completely dry.
- In a cast-iron skillet, heat bacon Fat and sear steaks for 1 minute per side.
- Serve steaks alongside Brussels sprouts.

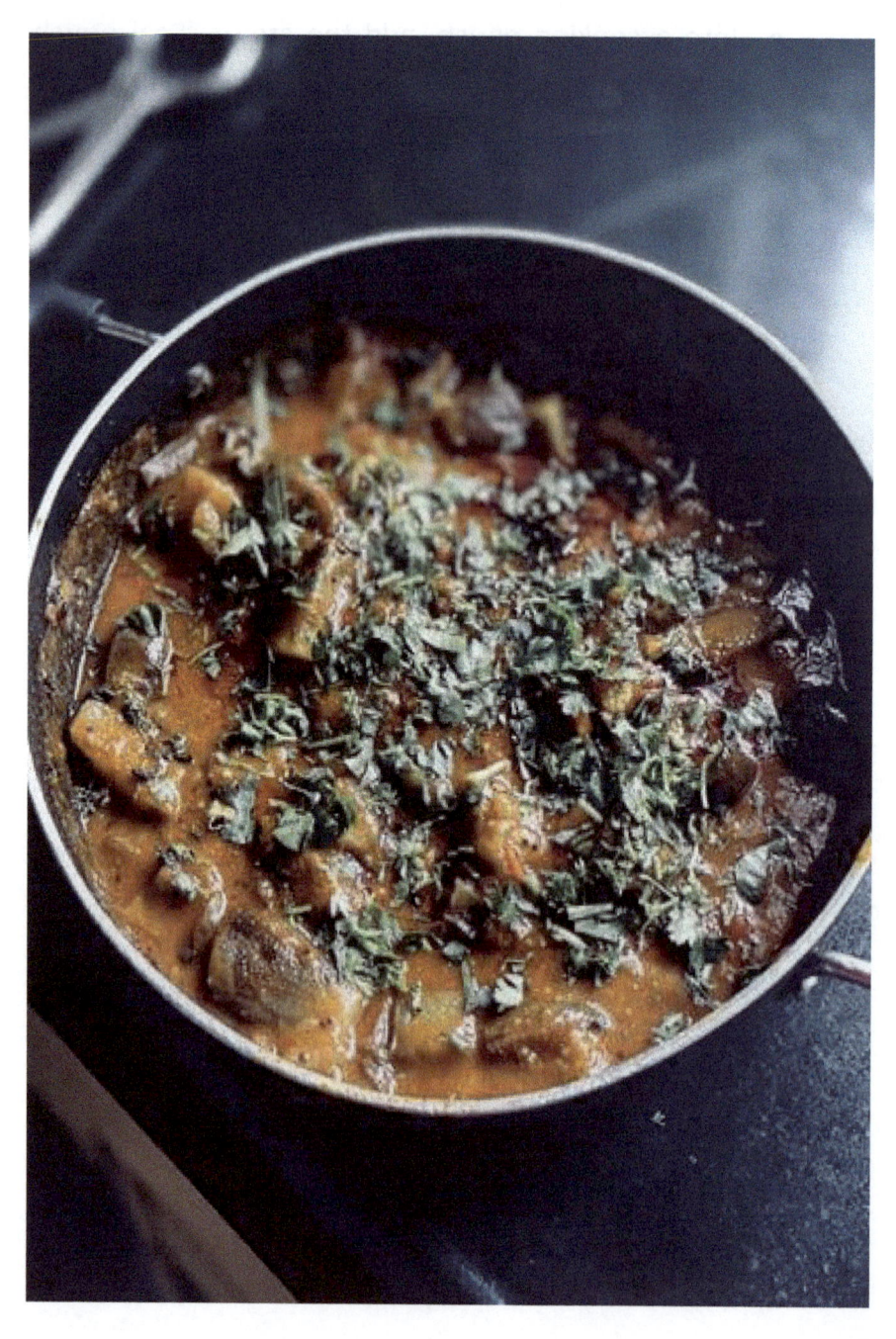

Lamb Steaks

4 Servings

Preparation Time: 6 hours 10 minutes

Ingredients:

- ⅔ cup olive oil, divided as ½ cup and the remaining oil
- 4 garlic cloves, crushed
- 1 sprig thyme
- 1 sprig rosemary
- 1 bay leaf
- 4 x 7-ounce lamb leg steaks

Directions:

- In a large bowl, mix together ½ cup of oil, garlic, the herbs and the bay leaf.
- Add steaks to bowl and coat generously with mixture.
- Refrigerate for 1-4 hours.
- Attach the sous vide immersion circulator using an adjustable clamp to a Cambro container or pot filled with water and preheat to 144°F.

- Into a cooking pouch, add steaks and remaining oil. Seal pouch tightly after squeezing out the excess air. Place pouch in sous vide bath and set the cooking time for 6 hours.
- Remove pouch from sous vide bath and carefully open it. Remove steaks from pouch. With paper towels, pat steaks completely dry.
- Heat a cast iron skillet over high heat, and sear steaks until browned from both sides.
- Serve immediately.

Lamb Sweetbreads

4 Servings

Preparation Time: 55 minutes

Ingredients:

- 4 cups milk, divided
- 10 ounces lamb sweetbreads
- 3 ½ ounces soft flour
- 1-ounce dried rosemary, crushed
- salt and freshly ground black pepper, to taste
- oil, as required

Directions:

- Into a large bowl, add 2 cups of milk and the lamb sweetbreads, and allow to soak for 8 hours.
- Attach the sous vide immersion circulator using an adjustable clamp to a Cambro container or pot filled with water and preheat to 144°F.
- Drain lamb sweetbreads.
- Into a large pan, add 4 cups of water and bring to a boil.
- Add lamb sweetbreads and cook for 10 seconds.

- Remove lamb sweetbreads from boiling water and immediately plunge into a large bowl of ice water to cool.
- After cooling, peel off any excess sinew.
- Into a cooking pouch, add lamb sweetbreads and the remaining 2 cups of milk. Seal pouch tightly after squeezing out the excess air. Place pouch in sous vide bath and set the cooking time for 40 minutes.
- Remove pouch from sous vide bath and carefully open it. Remove lamb sweetbreads from pouch. With paper towels, pat lamb sweetbreads completely dry.
- In a bowl, mix together the flour, rosemary, salt and black pepper.
- Roll lamb sweetbreads evenly with flour mixture.
- In a cast iron pan, heat some oil and fry and pan fry lamb sweetbreads until crisp.
- Serve immediately.

Venison Steaks

4 Servings

Preparation Time: 55 minutes

Ingredients:

For Steaks:

- 1 x 1-pound venison blade steak
- 2 shallots, roughly chopped
- 6 cloves garlic, roughly chopped
- 3 chili peppers, seeded and roughly chopped
- salt and freshly ground black pepper, to taste
- 1 tablespoon avocado oil

For Gravy:

- reserved cooking liquid mixture
- 2 tablespoons butter
- 1 teaspoon all-purpose flour
- 1 cup beef broth
- For Garnish:
- black mustard blossoms
- micro green herbs
- red amaranth

Directions:

- For the steak:
- To a large bowl, add the steak, shallots, garlic, chili peppers, salt, and pepper, and toss to coat well.
- Refrigerate for at least 30 minutes.
- Attach the sous vide immersion circulator using an adjustable clamp to a Cambro container or pot filled with water and preheat to 137°F.
- Into a cooking pouch, add steak mixture. Seal pouch tightly after squeezing out the excess air. Place pouch in sous vide bath and place a weight over pouch. Set the cooking time for 36 hours.
- Remove pouch from sous vide bath and carefully open it. Remove steak from pouch, reserving cooking liquid mixture. With paper towels, pat steak completely dry and set aside to rest briefly.
- In a skillet, heat 1 tablespoon of avocado oil and sear steak for 1 minute per side.
- Transfer steak onto a plate and keep aside.
- For the gravy:
- In a food processor, add the reserved cooking liquid mixture and pulse until a smooth paste is formed.
- In a heavy-bottomed pan, melt butter. Stir in flour and paste cook until browned slightly, stirring continuously.

- Reduce heat and stir in paste and broth. Bring to a boil and remove from heat.
- Cut steak into desired slices and decorate with favorite garnish.
- Serve with gravy.

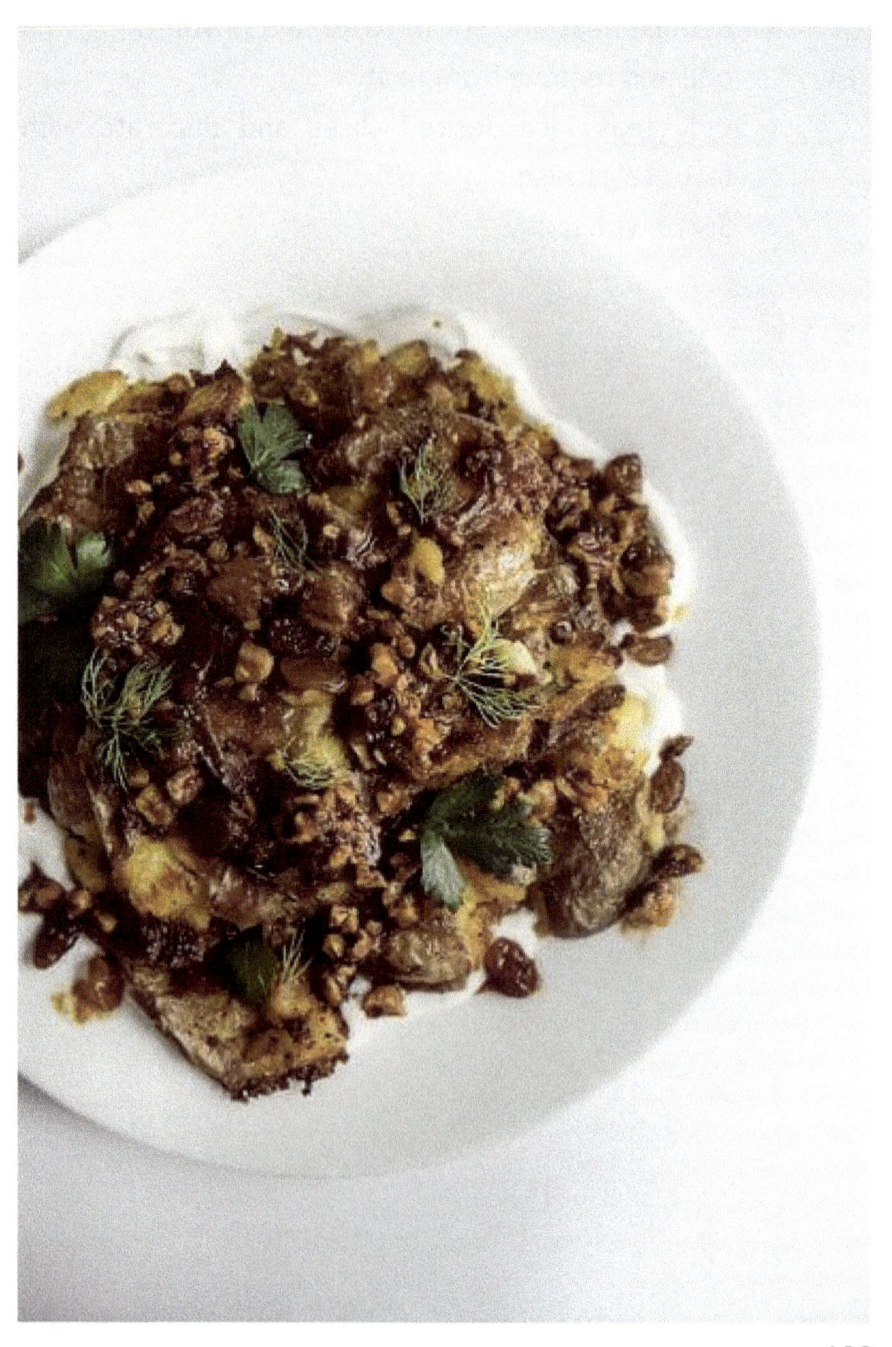

Osso Buco

4 Servings

Preparation Time: 72 hours 20 minutes

Ingredients:

- 2 veal shanks
- salt and freshly ground black pepper, to taste
- flour, as required
- extra-virgin olive oil, as required
- butter, as required
- 1 onion, chopped
- 2 ounces pancetta, chopped
- 1 glass dry white wine
- ½ cup concentrated veal broth
- 2 teaspoons tomato paste

For Gremolata:

- fresh flat leaf parsley, as required
- 1 fresh sprig rosemary
- 2 fresh sage leaves
- fresh lemon zest, as required
- 1 garlic clove

Directions:

- Attach the sous vide immersion circulator using an adjustable clamp to a Cambro container or pot filled with water and preheat to 143°F.
- With a sharp knife, make 1-inch cuts around the shanks.
- With paper towels, pat shanks and season with salt and black pepper.
- Dust each shank with flour evenly.
- In a frying pan, heat olive oil and sear shanks until browned from both sides.
- Transfer shanks onto a plate. Discard most of the oil from the pan.
- In the same pan, melt butter and sauté onion until translucent.
- Add pancetta and sauté until slightly golden.
- Stir in wine and cook until half the wine is absorbed.
- Stir in veal broth and tomato paste, then remove from heat.
- Into a large cooking ouch, place shanks and wine mixture. Seal pouch tightly after squeezing out the excess air. Place pouch in sous vide bath and set the cooking time for 72 hours.
- Meanwhile for gremolata:

- In a food processor, add all ingredients listed under gremolata section above, and pulse until minced finely.
- Remove pouch from sous vide bath and carefully open it. Remove shanks from pouch.
- Transfer shanks with mixture onto serving platter. Top with gremolata and serve.

Rabbit Loin

4 Servings

Preparation Time: 4 hours 20 minutes

Ingredients:

- 6 tablespoons olive oil, divided 4 + 2
- 1-ounce fresh flat leaf parsley, chopped
- ½ ounce fresh dill, chopped
- 2 tablespoons Dijon mustard
- 1 teaspoon apple cider vinegar
- 1 teaspoon garlic, minced
- ½ teaspoon freshly ground black pepper
- ¼ teaspoon ground ginger
- pinch of salt
- 4 x 8-ounce rabbit loins

Directions:

- Attach the sous vide immersion circulator using an adjustable clamp to a Cambro container or pot filled with water and preheat to 150°F.
- Into a bowl, add all ingredients except 2 tablespoons of oil and the rabbit loins. Mix well.

- Add rabbit loins and coat generously with mixture.
- In 4 separate cooking pouches, divide rabbit loins with marinade. Seal pouches tightly after squeezing out the excess air. Place pouches in sous vide bath and set the cooking time for 4 hours.
- Remove pouches from sous vide bath and carefully open them. Remove rabbit loins from pouches. With paper towels, pat rabbit loins completely dry.
- In a skillet, heat the remaining oil and sear the loins until golden brown from both sides.

DESSERT

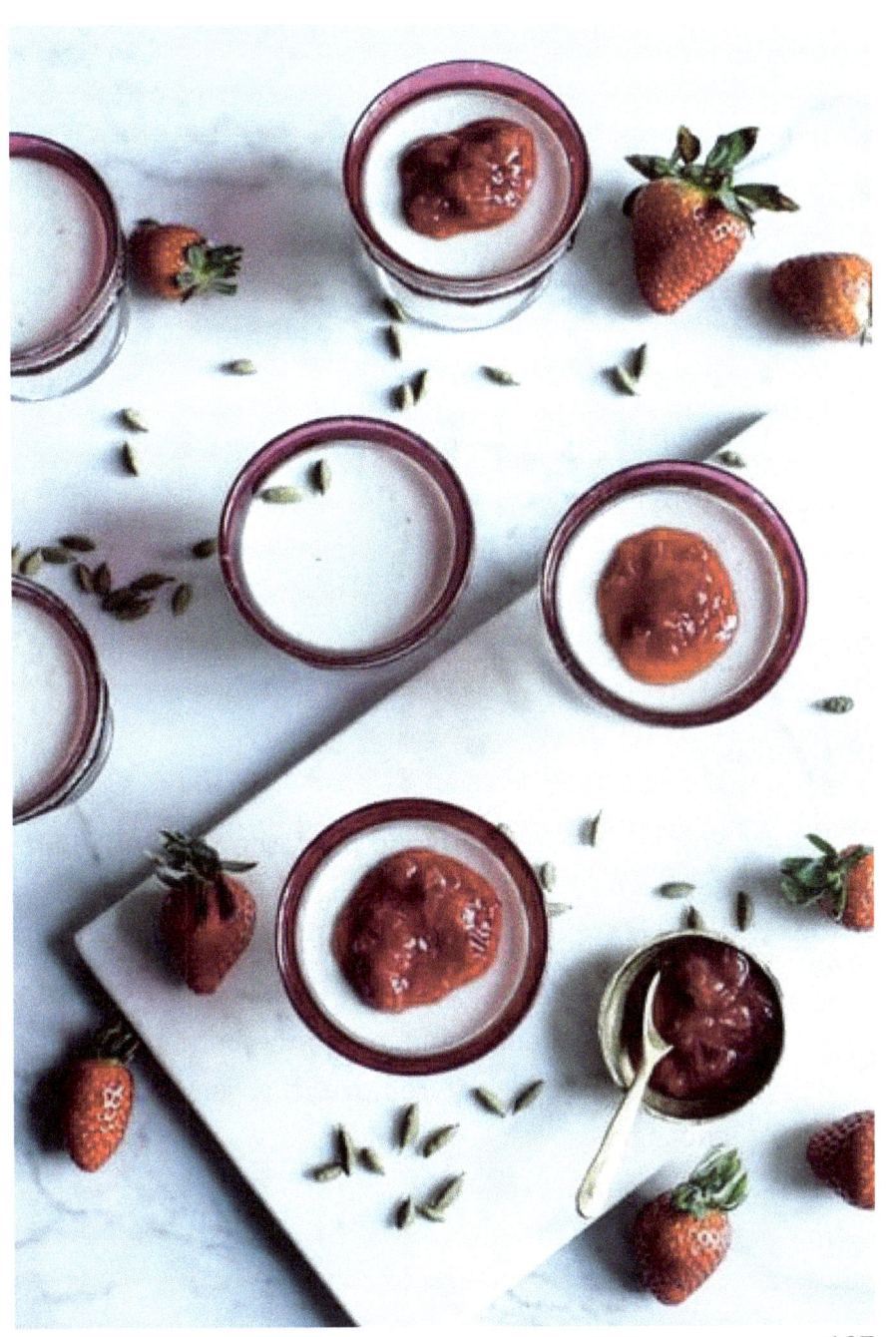

Vanilla Apricot Crumble

6 Servings

Preparation Time: 4 hours 15 minutes

Ingredients:

- 1 cup self-rising flour
- 1 cup granulated sugar
- 1 cup milk
- 1 tsp vanilla extract
- 8 tbsp melted butter
- 2 cups chopped apricots

Directions:

- Prepare a water bath and place the Sous Vide in it. Set to 194 F. Grease 6 canning jars with butter.
- Combine flour and sugar. Add in milk and vanilla. Mix in butter and apricots. Pour the mixture into the jars. Seal and submerge in the bath. Cook for 3 hours. Once done, remove the jars and allow cooling.
- Nutrition:

Savory Banana & Nuts Cups

12 Servings

Preparation Time: 3 hours 25 minutes

Ingredients:

- ½ cup butter
- ½ cup brown sugar
- ½ cup honey
- 2 eggs
- 1 tsp vanilla
- ½ tsp salt
- 3 tbsps milk
- 3 mashed bananas
- ½ tsp baking soda
- 2 cups all-purpose flour
- ½ cup nuts

Directions:

- Prepare a water bath and place the Sous Vide in it. Set to 172 F.
- Heat a pot over medium heat and cook the butter with the brown and white sugar. Remove from the

heat and allow cooling. Stir in the egg, vanilla, milk and honey. Cook until the sugar dissolved. Add the banana, flour, baking soda and salt. Mix well. Pour the mixture into mason jars. Seal and submerge the jars in the water bath. Cook for 2 hours.
- Once the timer has stopped, remove the jars and serve.

Orange Cheesy Mousse

8 Servings

Preparation Time: 2 hours 25 minutes

Ingredients:

- 2 cups milk
- 6 tbsps white wine vinegar
- 4 oz chocolate chips
- ¼ cup powdered sugar
- Grand Marnier liquor
- 1 tbsp orange zest
- 2 oz goat cheese

Directions:

- Prepare a water bath and place the Sous Vide in it. Set to 172 F.
- Place the milk and vinegar in a vacuum-sealable bag. Release air by the water displacement method, seal and submerge the bag in the water bath. Cook for 60 minutes.
- Once the timer has stopped, remove the bag and reserve the curds. Discard the remaining liquid.

Strain the curds for 10 minutes. Allow chilling for 1 hour.
- Prepare a water bath to medium heat and add the chocolate chips. Cook until melted. Transfer to a blender and stir the sugar, orange zest, grand Marnier, goat cheese. Mix until smooth. Serve into individual bowls.

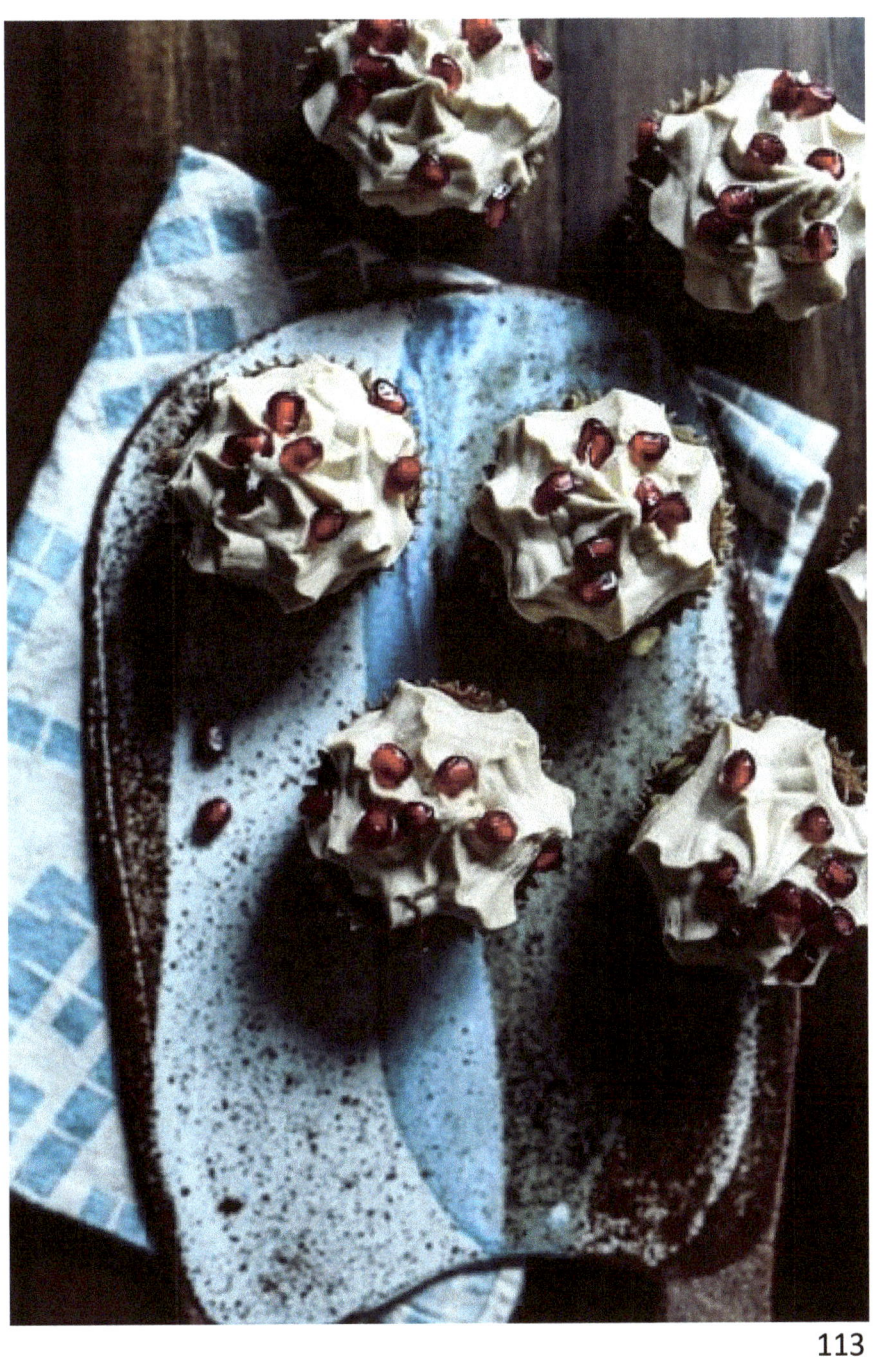

Coconut Blackberry Tart

4 Servings

Preparation Time: 2 hours 10 minutes

Ingredients:

- 1 egg
- ¼ cup heavy cream
- ¼ cup almond flour
- 1 tbsp sugar
- 2 tsps coconut flour
- ¼ tsp baking powder
- ¼ tsp vanilla extract
- ½ cup fresh blackberries
- Granulated sugar to garnish

Directions:

- Prepare a water bath and place the Sous Vide in it. Set to 186 F. Combine well all the Ingredients:, except the blackberries. Grease the mason jars with cooking spray and pour in the mixture. Top with 2 tbsps of blackberries each jar. Seal and submerge the jars in the water bath. Cook for 60 minutes.

- Once the timer has stopped, remove the jars.
- Garnish with sugar.

Lemon & Berry Mousse

8 Servings

Preparation Time: 1 hour 65 minutes

Ingredients:

- 1-pound raspberries, halved
- ¼ cup light brown sugar
- 3 tbsps freshly squeezed lemon juice
- ½ tsp salt
- ¼ tsp ground cinnamon
- 1 cup heavy cream
- 1 tsp vanilla extract
- 1 cup crème fraiche

Directions:

- Prepare a water bath and place the Sous Vide in it. Set to 182 F.
- Place the raspberries, brown sugar, lemon juice, salt and cinnamon in a vacuum-sealable bag. Release air by water displacement method, seal and submerge the bag in the water bath. Cook for 45 minutes.

- Once the timer has stopped, remove the bag and transfer the contents to a blender. Stir until smooth.
- Whisk the heavy cream and vanilla. Pour in the raspberries mix with the créme fraiche and combine well. Transfer into 8 serving bowls. Allow chilling.

Creamy Blueberry Mousse

8 Servings

Preparation Time: 2 hours

Ingredients:

- 1-pound blueberries
- ¼ cup sugar
- 3 tbsps lemon juice
- ¼ tsp ground cinnamon
- 1 cup heavy cream
- 1 tsp vanilla extract

Directions:

- Prepare a water bath and place the Sous Vide in it. Set to 182 F.
- Combine the blueberries, sugar, lemon juice and cinnamon and place in a vacuum-sealable bag. Release air by the water displacement method, seal and submerge the bag in the water bath. Cook for 30 minutes.

- Once ready, remove the bag and transfer the contents to a blender. Stir until smooth. Whisk the cream and vanilla. Pour in the blueberries mix and combine well. Transfer into 8 serving bowls. Allow chilling.

Fruity Chocolate Flan

12 Servings

Preparation Time: 5 hours 50 minutes

Ingredients:

- 1 cup fruit-forward red wine
- ½ cup granulated sugar
- 12 oz white chocolate chips
- 8 oz white chocolate, chopped
- 1 cup milk
- ½ cup heavy cream
- 8 egg yolks

Directions:

- Prepare a water bath and place the Sous Vide in it. Set to 182 F.
- Heat a saucepan over medium heat and pour the wine and sugar. Stir for 20 minutes until reduced. Allow cooling for 10 minutes. Transfer to a blender and put the chocolate chips, milk, cream, and egg yolks. Mix until smooth.
- Place the mixture in a vacuum-sealable bag. Release air by the water

- Displacement method, seal and submerge the bag in the water bath. Cook for 45 minutes. Once the timer has stopped, remove the bag and transfer the contents to a blender and mix for 2 minutes. Share into 12 ramekins and cover with plastic.
- Allow chilling for 4 hours and serve.

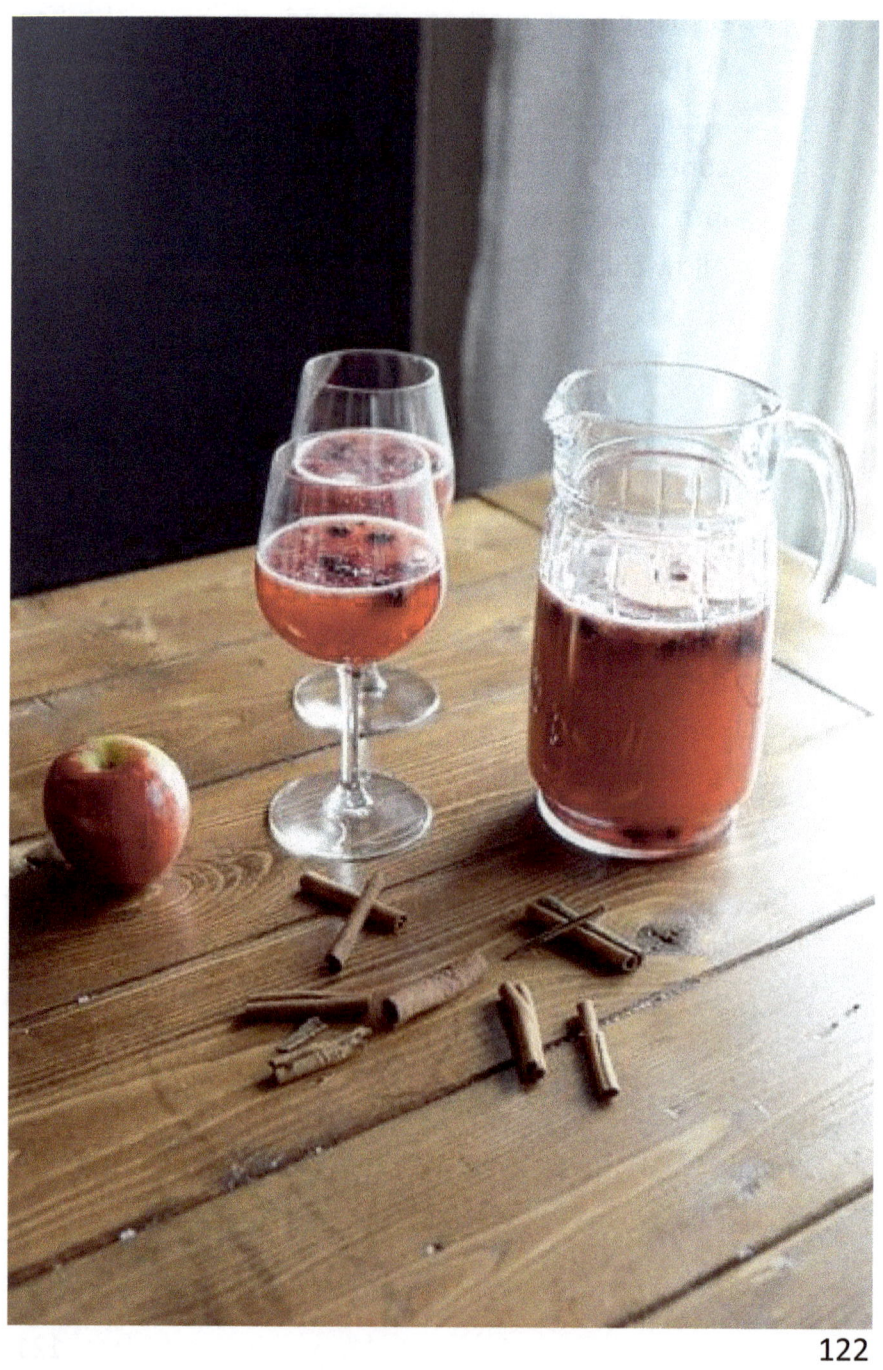

Maple Lemon Brioche Pudding

4 Servings

Preparation Time: 3 hours 20 minutes

Ingredients:

- 1 cup whole milk
- 1 cup heavy cream
- ½ cup granulated sugar
- ¼ cup maple syrup
- 2 tbsps lemon juice
- 1 tbsp lemon zest
- 1 tsp vanilla bean paste
- 4 cups brioche, cubed

Directions:

- Prepare a water bath and place the Sous Vide in it. Set to 172 F.
- Combine well the milk, heavy cream, sugar, maple syrup, lemon zest, lemon juice, vanilla bean paste.
- Put the brioche and mix together.

- Pour the mixture into 4 mason jars.
- Seal and submerge the jars in the water bath. Cook for 2 hours.
- Once the timer has stopped, remove the jars and transfer to the broiler.
- Bake for 2-3 minutes and serve

Lightning Source UK Ltd.
Milton Keynes UK
UKHW021101220721
387582UK00001B/51